# Palliative care consultations in advanced breast cancer

# Palliative care consultations in advanced breast cancer

Edited by

## Sara Booth

Macmillan Consultant in Palliative Medicine,
Lead Clinician in Palliative Care,
Cambridge University Hospitals NHS Foundation Trust;
Honorary Senior Lecturer,
Department of Palliative Care and Policy,
King's College, London

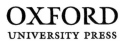

OXFORD
UNIVERSITY PRESS

# OXFORD
UNIVERSITY PRESS

Great Clarendon Street, Oxford OX2 6DP

Oxford University Press is a department of the University of Oxford.
It furthers the University's objective of excellence in research, scholarship,
and education by publishing worldwide in

Oxford New York

Auckland Cape Town Dar es Salaam Hong Kong Karachi
Kuala Lumpur Madrid Melbourne Mexico City Nairobi
New Delhi Shanghai Taipei Toronto

With offices in

Argentina Austria Brazil Chile Czech Republic France Greece
Guatemala Hungary Italy Japan Poland Portugal Singapore
South Korea Switzerland Thailand Turkey Ukraine Vietnam

Oxford is a registered trade mark of Oxford University Press
in the UK and in certain other countries

Published in the United States
by Oxford University Press Inc., New York

A catalogue record for this title is available from the British Library

Library of Congress Cataloging in Publication Data

Palliative care consultations in advanced breast cancer/edited by Sara Booth.
    p.;cm.— (Palliative care consultations)
    Includes bibliographical references and index.
    1. Breast—Cancer—Palliative treatment. 2. Breast—Cancer—Complications.
I. Booth, Sara, Dr. II. Series.

[DNLM: 1. Breast Neoplasms—therapy. 2. Breast Neoplasms—complication. 3. Palliative
Care—methods.    WP 870 P164 2006]
RC280.B8P25 2006
616.99'44906—dc22

                                                      2005019521

Typeset by SPI Publisher Services, Pondicherry, India
Printed in Great Britain
on acid-free paper by Biddles Ltd., King's Lynn

ISBN 0-19-853075-7 (pbk: alk.paper) 978–019–853075–6

10 9 8 7 6 5 4 3 2 1

# Series Foreword

Despite the significant advances in diagnosis and treatment that have been made in recent decades, cancer remains a major cause of death in all developed countries. It is therefore essential that all health professionals who provide direct care for cancer patients should be aware of what can be done to alleviate suffering.

Major progress has been made over the past thirty years or so in the relief of physical symptoms and in approaches to the delivery of psychological, social, and spiritual care for cancer patients and their families and carers. However, the problems of providing holistic care should not be underestimated. This is particularly the case in busy acute general hospitals and cancer centres. The physical environment may not be conducive to the care of a dying patient. Staff may have difficulty recognizing the point at which radical interventions are no longer in a patient's best interests, when the emphasis should change to care with palliative intent.

Progress in the treatment of cancer has also led to many patients who, although incurable, living for years with their illness. They may have repeated courses of treatment and some will have a significant burden of symptoms that must be optimally controlled.

One of the most important developments in recent years has been the recognition of the benefits of a multidisciplinary or multiprofessional approach to cancer care. Physicians, surgeons, radiologists, haematologists, pathologists, oncologists, palliative care specialists, nurse specialists, and a wide range of other health professionals all have major contributions to make. These specialists need to work together in teams.

One of the prerequisites for effective teamwork is that individual members should recognize the contribution that others can make. The *Palliative Care Consultations* series should help to make this a reality. The editors are to be congratulated in bringing together distinguished cancer and palliative care specialists from all parts of the world. Individual volumes focus predominantly on the problems faced by patients with a particular type of cancer (e.g. breast or lung) or groups of cancers (e.g. haematological malignancies or gynaecological cancers). The chapters of each volume set out what can be achieved using anticancer treatments and through the delivery of palliative care.

I warmly welcome the series and I believe the individual volumes will prove valuable to a wide range of clinicians involved in the delivery of high quality care.

Professor M A Richards
National Cancer Director, England

# Preface

Many aspects of the oncological and palliative care management of breast cancer exemplify some significant cultural changes and medical advances that have taken place in the last fifty years.

Cancer was once a 'taboo' subject – patients even felt a sense of shame on learning that they had the disease, it could not be named. The suffering felt by those who felt they had to conceal the illness, or had it concealed from them, can only be imagined. Treatment was once surgery alone, then the advance of radiotherapy was added to primary treatment. Both were mutilating and onerous and if they did not cure, the disease would kill, often quickly and painfully. It was usual for patients to be told what was best for them and it was a rare woman who demurred. The adverse effects of early chemotherapy regimens could not be controlled easily and after intensive treatment had been given there were no palliative treatments.

Breast cancer is now possibly the 'most talked about' cancer in everyday life: it is so common that most people know someone close to them, perhaps a relative, friend, neighbour or colleague who has been affected. It receives attention in the media because of medical advances in treatment, or less happily because of failures and perceived failures in management by individual doctors, other clinicians or health care systems. More positively, many women who have experienced breast cancer tell their stories in local and national newspapers, books and daytime and mainstream slots on television, and inspire and inform other sufferers. Major charities like Cancer Relief Macmillan, 'Breakthrough Breast Cancer' and many others have publicised the needs of women with breast cancer. The unmentionable, even thirty years ago, has become the topic of everyday conversations and whilst many people still 'don't know what to say' when someone close tells them she has breast cancer, they often know a bit about the experience their friend or relative is going through, that she will need emotional support as well as medical treatment, and where she can go for help. Cancer is now *mentionable* and although the feeling of being stigmatised still affects many patients with all cancers, this has reduced in incidence and enabled many more people living with cancer to ask for the help they need.

Naturally perhaps, the public emphasis is on the women who are cured, and advances in oncology mean that this has become much more common. The public perception of breast cancer is therefore changing to that of a curable illness. In all this, the advances in the management of advanced cancer should not be overlooked, as they too are hopeful for those with metastatic disease.

Now it may be possible for an individual to live longer with advanced disease and experience a good quality of life with relatively benign palliative oncological treatments, some being given in tablet form. This has meant that many cancer patients now live with a chronic illness, which requires a different outlook to an immediately life-threatening one. Oncologists are now starting to set up systems to give 'supportive care' to help those patients who could otherwise live from the time of diagnosis mostly asymptomatically, but with the possibility of a constant background threat shadowing their lives – unless they get the help they need to contain it. Other patients could live for months, perhaps years, with intrusive symptoms – the disease always a reality for them without effective symptom control.

These changes in oncology treatment and outlook have brought about a change in the way palliative care physicians work with their colleagues in oncology: it is no longer an 'over to you' one way journey from oncology to palliative care, common in the 1980s and early 1990s. Working in partnership with the patient and his/her carers to give palliative oncological therapy in conjunction with palliative care is the usual pattern now. Palliative care teams may see a patient during a symptomatic spell, then not see the patient for months or years. Rehabilitation and long-term support, both physical and psychological, is becoming increasingly important in oncology and palliative care management. Many patients want to play a very active part in the decisions concerning their treatment. Palliative care clinicians recognize that palliative endocrine and chemotherapy are usually relatively easy to undergo and can be integrated into a full active life and reduce symptoms. Targeted biological treatments such as Herceptin may be leading the way in an exciting new therapeutic direction for advanced disease.

These issues are discussed in depth in the first and third chapters. The care of the patient who lives with long-term symptoms and the complications of advanced disease are discussed in the chapters on lymphoedema, fatigue, bisphosphonates and bone metastases.

Breast cancer, however, remains a disease that can kill young people quickly and painfully, and one that can present late in older women who may conceal an obvious cancer until it becomes too malodorous or disseminated to hide any longer. There are separate chapters to cover the subjects of pain in advanced local disease, carcinomatous meningitis and odours and wounds: they are difficult and demanding problems to treat and there is little evidence from controlled trials to aid clinicians and patients. The book finishes with a review of the management of pleural effusions – common and very disabling - and an area where there have been important advances in recent years.

This book was planned with Eduardo Bruera who has also co-authored an outstanding chapter on the management of the complications of bone metastases. His famously busy schedule meant that he had to step down from co-editing. I am very grateful for his interest and support in the early stages. Helena Earl has been a thoughtful and active specialist co-editor and I would like to thank her – she has also co-authored an authoritative first chapter illustrated with moving case histories.

All the contributors have been committed and enthusiastic and I would like to acknowledge their work – they are all obviously very dedicated to their patients and their special interest, and it is clear why the management of metastatic disease is advancing at a rapid pace. We would all like to see all cancers cured, and an end to the suffering of advanced disease, but whilst it is with us, we need to understand how best to help our patients. This book was commissioned to give you that information. It has been both a great pleasure and an education to work with all the authors. I hope that you enjoy reading it and find what you need for your clinical practice within.

Sara Booth
August 2005

# Contents

# Contributors

**Athar Ahmad**, Consultant in Medical Oncology, Queen Elizabeth Hospital, Kings Lynn; Addenbrooke's Hospital, Cambridge, UK

**Angela Bentley**, Specialist Registrar in Palliative Medicine, Western General Hospital, Edinburgh, UK

**Eduardo Bruera**, Professor of Palliative Medicine, University of Texas M.D. Anderson Cancer Center, Houston, Texas, USA

**Helena Earl**, Lecturer and Honorary Consultant in Medical Oncology, University of Cambridge Department of Oncology, Addenbrooke's Hospital, Cambridge, UK

**Marie Fallon**, Senior Lecturer, University of Edinburgh; Honorary Consultant, Department of Palliative Medicine, Western General Hospital, Edinburgh, UK

**Christina Faull**, Consultant in Palliative Medicine, University Hospitals of Leicester and the Leicestershire and Rutland Hospice; Honorary Senior Lecturer, University of Leicester, UK

**Kathryn G. Froiland**, Oncology Clinical Educator, GlaxoSmithKline Inc, Houston, Texas, USA

**Elizabeth A. Grunfeld**, Senior Lecturer, Section of Health Psychology, Institute of Psychiatry, King's College London, UK

**Mahesh Iddawela**, Specialist Registrar in Medical Oncology, Addenbrooke's Hospital, Cambridge, UK

**Anil A. Joy**, Medical Oncologist, Cross Cancer Institute; Assistant Professor, Department of Oncology, University of Alberta, Edmonton, Canada

**Benedict Konzen**, Assistant Professor, Department of Palliative Care and Rehabilitation Medicine, University of Texas M.D. Anderson Cancer Center, Houston, Texas, USA

**John R. Mackey**, Medical Oncologist, Cross Cancer Institute; Associate Professor, Department of Oncology, University of Alberta, Edmonton, Canada

**Karen McAdam**, Consultant in Medical Oncology, Peterborough Hospital Foundation Trust; Addenbrooke's Hospital, Cambridge, UK

**Scott A. North**, Medical Oncologist, Cross Cancer Institute; Associate Professor, Department of Oncology, University of Alberta, Edmonton, Canada

**A.H.G. Paterson**, Tom Baker Cancer Centre; Professor, University of Calgary, Alberta, Canada

**Ki Y. Shin**, Assistant Professor and Section Chief, Department of Palliative Care and Rehabilitation Medicine, University of Texas M.D. Anderson Cancer Center, Houston, Texas, USA

**Catherine Sweeney**, Medical Tutor, Marymount Hospice, St Patrick's Hospital, Cork, Ireland

**Gillian Whitfield**, Specialist Registrar in Clinical Oncology, Addenbooke's Hospital, Cambridge, UK

**Yolanda Zuriarrain Reyna**, Palliative Care Physician, Centro de Cuidados Paliativos Laguna, Madrid, Spain

Chapter 1

# Current management of advanced breast cancer

Mahesh Iddawela, Athar Ahmad, Karen McAdam, and Helena Earl

## Summary

At the point of development of metastatic disease, breast cancer is defined as incurable. The aims of therapy then change to keeping the patient '*as well as possible for as long as possible*'. This implies that prolongation of life is important despite the impossibility of cure, but that attention to quality of life and therefore side-effects of treatment plays an equally important part. In many ways this has become the '*art of oncology*'. In breast cancer, response rates to treatment are so high that '*active palliative anticancer treatment*' with hormonal and chemotherapy is universally accepted as the best way to both prolong life and improve its quality. The first decision for the oncologists is whether to use hormonal treatment or chemotherapy. Hormone receptor status in the primary breast cancer guides decisions here. It is more difficult at present to quantify clinical judgements concerning chemotherapy and they remain largely in the sphere of *qualitative decision-making*. In other words the oncologist has to develop expertise and make clinical judgements about what treatment to give, how much, when to start, how long to carry on, in what order to give active agents, and whether to combine drugs together to achieve higher response rates at the cost of greater toxicity. There will still be a few patients in whom treatment is inappropriate, and palliative and supportive care are the best options from the outset. In our opinion and that of many UK breast cancer specialists, there is a real need to develop better prognostic and predictive markers of response to different therapies. There is also a need to evolve clinical trials in the metastatic setting which will begin to answer some of the questions outlined above, which remain so important for women who have the misfortune to develop metastatic breast cancer. Newer 'targeted' agents, such as herceptin, offer great hope in this field, since they will target tumours and produce less toxicity, thus fulfilling the stated aim: *to keep women with metastatic breast cancer as well as possible for as long as possible*.

## Introduction

Breast cancer is the most common solid tumour in women in the US and Western Europe. Its incidence has increased considerably over the past 10 years and approximately 40 000 cases of breast cancer are now diagnosed each year in the UK. Although cure rates have also risen because of better local and systemic treatment in the early stages of the disease, the number of women diagnosed and living with metastatic breast cancer remains very high.[1] Hence the importance of the management of metastatic breast cancer as a topic for this series, Palliative Care Consultations. Many treatments are available, which include systemic chemotherapy and hormone therapy, palliative radiotherapy and newer 'biological' therapies, the most successful of which to date has proved to be herceptin, a monoclonal antibody. These have response rates that lead to significant palliation of cancer symptoms and prolongation of life for women with metastatic disease. 'Active' palliative treatment, which makes significant use of increasingly available systemic treatments, is a vital part of palliative management of women with metastatic breast cancer.

The median survival for metastatic breast cancer patients is 2–3 years but disease burden and number of sites of metastatic disease affect this. Patients with non-visceral disease have a median survival of 40 months but for those with visceral disease it is about 18–24 months. At the time of relapse the aim of treatment is palliation of symptoms first and prolongation of life second. Hence the toxicity of treatment and its impact on quality of life are important factors, which need to be carefully considered. There is emerging evidence that the overall survival of metastatic or locally advanced breast cancer is improving due to the introduction of better treatments. A retrospective study, looking at patients with metastatic breast cancer treated at a single institution, showed that patients presenting between 1974 and 1979 had a median survival of 15 months, whereas patients developing metastatic disease between 1995 and 2000 had a median survival of 51 months.[2] A further population-based study in Canada demonstrated that the advent of new therapies during the 1990s led to a significant improvement in overall survival for patients treated in the latter part of the decade.[3]

Common sites of breast cancer metastasis can be divided into two major categories: loco-regional (chest wall, axilla, or supraclavicular metastasis) or distant (lung, liver, bone, and brain). Patients with locally advanced breast cancers which are not surgically resectable can be treated with neoadjuvant therapy, which includes both endocrine treatment and chemotherapy. Treatment of these patients follows a similar pattern to treatment of metastatic disease, although radical radiotherapy and palliative surgery also play a role.

## Management

### Treatment options

When a patient develops metastatic disease, several factors govern the decisions about the optimal treatment for that individual; these include: age, menopausal status, sites of metastases, oestrogen receptor (ER) status, human epidermal growth factor-2 over-expression, and time to the development of first metastasis (disease-free interval). One important decision that has to be made early is whether the patient (if ER positive) can have a trial of hormonal treatment first, or should start immediately on chemotherapy. If the patient has ER-negative breast cancer, then endocrine therapy is not an option.

Very few women with metastatic breast cancer (less than 20%) achieve a complete response to treatment. The majority of patients on treatment achieve a partial response or stable disease. Stabilization of disease is an important end point as it halts the worsening of symptoms and thus maintains the quality of life of the patient. The better the response to endocrine or chemotherapy the longer the treatment-free interval, with patients who do achieve a complete response having the longest disease-free and overall survival.

## Endocrine therapy

Endocrine therapy was established as an important modality of treatment for metastatic breast cancer as long ago as 1896, when Beatson described the regression of skin metastases in women who had been treated by oophorectomy.[4] Unless there is life-threatening visceral disease (liver, lung, and brain) and rapid response is required, systemic hormonal therapy is preferred first-line therapy in metastatic disease which is ER-positive (Fig. 1.1). Relative to chemotherapy, this treatment has low toxicity and around 40–60% of ER-positive patients will respond. When progesterone receptors (PR) are also positive in the primary tumour the response rate increases to 60–80%. In the uncommon scenario of ER-negative but PR-positive breast cancer, there can be up to 30% response rate to endocrine therapy.

Factors that predict endocrine responsiveness include postmenopausal status, older age, good performance status, human epidermal growth factor negativity (HER-2 negative), and long interval between diagnosis and the development of metastases.

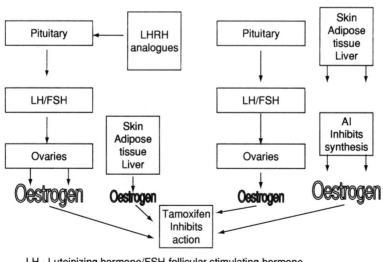

LH - Luteinizing hormone/FSH-follicular stimulating hormone
LHRH - luteinizing hormone releasing hormone
AI - aromatase inhibitor

**Fig. 1.1** Mechanism of action of hormonal treatment for breast cancer.

The treatment is for those without rapidly progressive disease and minimal/ moderate disease burden.

Metastatic breast cancer patients with bone-only metastases, soft tissue disease (e.g. axillary or supraclavicular lymphadenopathy, skin metastases), or asymptomatic visceral metastases are candidates for first-line endocrine treatment. Meta-analysis of patients with visceral disease on trials of anastrazole has shown that there was no significant difference in time to progression. Although there are multiple agents, there is no evidence that combination hormonal treatment produces a survival advantage over sequential therapy even though combination regimens are associated with higher toxicity.

First-line endocrine treatment for postmenopausal women with metastatic breast cancer is with an aromatase inhibitor (AI) (anastrazole or letrozole) (Fig. 1.2). Compared to tamoxifen these agents have higher response rates, better tolerability, and lower incidence of thromboembolic episodes, although there is a higher incidence of osteoporosis and fractures.

Patients who fail on the first AI can be changed to another agent, so exemestane is used on failure of treatment with either anastrazole or letrozole. When these patients have progressed through the aromatase inhibitors, they can be changed to pure oestrogen antagonists such as fulvestran. Patients who progress on these agents, can receive progestins (such as megesterol acetate or medroxyprogesterone), if they remain candidates for further treatment.

There are few side-effects associated with endocrine therapy but as patients progress through multiple treatment modalities, the morbidity from the disease increases and the toxicity of even the endocrine therapy becomes significant. It is important for the multidisciplinary team managing the patient to discuss and re-establish the aims of

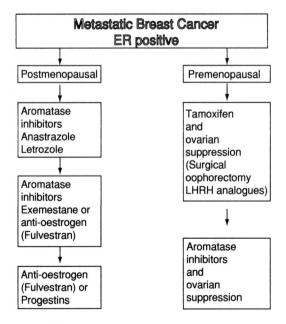

**Fig. 1.2** Treatment algorithm.

management, as at some point in the patient pathway the best option will become good palliative care without the use of active systemic therapy.

Letrozole (Femara®), was initially shown to be superior to megesterol acetate in the second-line treatment of advanced breast cancer as it produced a higher response rate and a longer duration of response. A randomized phase III trial comparing tamoxifen and letrozole in metastatic breast cancer patients showed that the response to letrozole was superior to tamoxifen and the time to progression (TTP) was prolonged by 3.4 months (9.4 for letrozole against 6 months for tamoxifen).[5] There was a reduced incidence of thromboembolic events compared to tamoxifen (1% compared to 2%).

## Aromatase inhibitors

Aromatase inhibitors block the conversion of adrenal androgens to oestrogen in liver, muscle, and adipose tissue by the enzyme aromatase (cytochrome p450 enzymes). Aminoglutethemide was one of the first AIs used clinically but has been superseded by the new more potent and specific blockers which have a better toxicity profile (Table 1.1). These agents produce more than 90% reduction in the circulating oestrone and oestradiol.

Anastrazole was initially shown to be as effective as megesterol acetate in second-line treatment and has subsequently been shown to be as effective as tamoxifen in the first-line treatment of metastatic breast cancer. The reported response rates and the median TTP were similar when tamoxifen and anastrazole were compared but the toxicity profile of anastrazole was better with lower incidence of thromboembolic events and frequency of vaginal bleeding.[6]

Exemestane can be used as second-line hormonal therapy following failure of non-steroidal AI. When exemestane was compared with megestrol acetate in the second-line treatment of hormonal therapy, response rates were not significantly superior.[7] However, when exemestane was compared with tamoxifen, there was a superior response rate and a longer progression-free survival with exemestane. Steroidal AIs have a similar structure to the substrate of the aromatase enzyme and they bind to the enzyme irreversibly. This may produce some activity for exemestane after other AIs have stopped being effective.

**Table 1.1** Aromatase inhibitors

| Aromatase inhibitor | Nature of aromatase inhibition | Response compared to tamoxifen | Toxicity |
|---|---|---|---|
| **Non-steroidal** | | | |
| Letrozole | Competitive | 32% vs. 21% | Bone pain, hot flushes, nausea, fatigue |
| Anastrazole | Competitive | 32.9% vs. 32.6% | Hot flushes, nausea, asthenia |
| **Steroidal** | | | |
| Exemestane | Non-competitive | 44.2% vs. 29.2% | Fatigue, hot flushes, nausea, pain |

Fulvestran is a specific antioestrogen with high affinity to ER without the disadvantages of agonist activity associated with tamoxifen (so it would not have any effects on the uterus). It is a novel agent that causes down-regulation of ER by binding to receptors. When anastrazole was compared to fulvestrant, in the first or second-line setting, there was no difference in the time to progression (TTP: 5.1 months vs. 5.5 months, respectively) or overall response rate (ORR: 15.7% and 20.7%, respectively). The most commonly reported side-effects are hot flushes, nausea, headache, and asthenia.[8]

## Progestins and tamoxifen

Following failure of AI and antioestrogens, if the patient is candidate for hormonal therapy, megesterol acetate or tamoxifen can be considered as there is some evidence that these agents can be effective at this stage.

## Management of premenopausal women

Tamoxifen (selective oestrogen receptor modulator (SERM)) and ovarian suppression are used as first-line therapy for metastatic breast cancer in premenopausal women. Ovarian suppression either with luteinizing hormone releasing hormone (LHRH) analogues such as Zoladex® or surgical oopherectomy have similar efficacy in dramatically lowering the circulating oestrogen levels. The meta-analysis of all trials comparing ovarian suppression alone with ovarian suppression and tamoxifen has shown a statistically significant advantage for combination therapy. The ORR was 29% for LHRH analogue alone and 38% for combination therapy with LHRH and tamoxifen. The median survival for the combination arm was 2.9 years and 2.5 years for LHRH analogues alone and was statistically significant.[9] This has established combination therapy as standard of care in premenopausal women. Patients progressing after these treatments can go onto AI as well, provided they are still on LHRH analogues or have had a surgical oophorectomy.

## Tamoxifen or oestrogen deprivation?

There is emerging evidence that tailoring endocrine therapy would form an important part in optimizing the benefit from treatment. There is evidence from *in vitro* and clinical trials that human epidermal receptor-2 over-expressing breast cancers are more responsive to aromatase inhibitors than tamoxifen.[10] In a neoadjuvant trial of primary endocrine therapy, the response rate was greater in HER-2 positive patients treated with letrozole than those treated with tamoxifen. This finding awaits validation in larger trials.

# Chemotherapy

For patients who progress on endocrine treatment or those with symptomatic visceral disease chemotherapy is the treatment of choice. Those who benefit from chemotherapy would obtain a response within 8–12 weeks and median duration of response varies between 5 and 15 months. Most responses to chemotherapy are partial and less than 20% of the patients will have a complete response. This is an important subset as several studies have reported a favourable prognosis for those achieving a complete response.

The standard chemotherapy for metastatic breast cancer has passed through several changes since it was introduced in the 1960s. Initially, single agents were used but the responses were short-lived. Combination regimens, such as cyclophosphamide, methotrexate and 5-flourouracil (CMF) and CMF plus prednisolone and vincristine, were introduced subsequently. These regimens demonstrated substantial activity but with the introduction of anthracyclines, which have similar single-agent activity to multidrug regimens, meant that single-agent anthracycline became commonplace in the 1980s.[11]

Combination chemotherapy has a higher response rate and a longer time to disease progression but only few trials have shown a significant survival advantage and it is associated with higher toxicity compared to sequential single-agent treatment.[11] The overall survival benefit from combination chemotherapy is small and tailoring of treatment to the needs and the fitness of the patient is one of the most important aspects of management. Those patients who are fit and value the small survival advantage that combination chemotherapy offers should be offered this, while those who are interested in maintaining their quality of life should have sequential single-agent treatment.

As adjuvant chemotherapy has become much more commonplace and as anthracycline-based chemotherapies have become standard, the majority of patients who develop metastatic disease would have had prior exposure and would be classified as resistant to anthracyclines. The first-line treatment for these patients is either a single agent taxane or taxane-containing combination (with epirubicin or herceptin).

## Single-agent chemotherapy

### Anthracyclines

Anthracyclines (doxorubicin and epirubicin) are one of the most effective classes of agents in metastatic breast cancer with response rates of 40–50%.[12] These agents can be given at lower doses on a weekly rather than a 3-weekly schedule; this is well tolerated and has been extensively used in frail patients with poor performance status. The drug is predominantly metabolized in the liver and, as a result, careful dose modification according to the liver function is important, especially when the bilirubin is elevated. Common side-effects are listed in Table 1.2. There is an exponential increase in the risk of cardiac toxicity above 450 mg/m$^2$ in the case of doxorubicin and 900 mg/m$^2$ with epirubicin. Most oncologists prefer epirubicin because of the lower gastrointestinal toxicity and higher cumulative dose required before cardiac function is affected.[13]

### Taxanes

These are derived from the Pacific yew tree (Paclitaxel®) or the European yew tree (Docetaxel®) and have response rates from 50–60% for docetaxel and 40–60% for paclitaxel. Importantly, both these agents are active in anthracycline pretreated patients. A trial comparing docetaxel with mitomycin and vinblastine (MV) has shown a significantly higher response rate to docetaxel (30% vs. 11.6%; p <0.001).

**Table 1.2** Common chemotherapy agents used in the management of metastatic breast cancer

| Drug | Dose/ route | Action | RR (%) | Side-effects |
|---|---|---|---|---|
| Doxorubicin | 60–70 mg/m$^2$ in every 3 weeks | DNA covalent bonds: topo-II inhibitor | 40–50 | N and V, myelosupression, stomatitis, cardiac toxicity |
| Epirubicin | 60–90 mg/m$^2$ iv every 3 weeks | DNA covalent bonds: topo-II inhibitor | 40–50 | N and V, myelosupression, stomatitis, cardiac toxicity |
| Paclitaxel | 135–175 mg/m$^2$ iv every 3 weeks | Inhibits microtubule complex assembly by tubulin polymerization | 40–60 | N and V, skin rashes, alopecia, peripheral neuropathy, arthalgias, myalgias, hypersensitivity reactions, myelosupression |
| Docetaxel | 75–100 mg/m$^2$ in every 3 weeks | Inhibits microtubule complex assembly by tubulin polymerization | 50–60 | N and V, myelosupression, skin rashes, nail changes, alopecia, peripheral neuropathy, hypersensitivity reactions, fluid retention/ pleural effusions |
| Capecitabine | 800–1250 mg/m$^2$ bd for 10–14 days | Metabolized to intermediates that inhibit DNA or RNA synthesis | 15–26 | Palmar plantar erythema, diarrhoea, stomatitis, V, fatigue |
| Gemcitabine | 1 gm/m$^2$ days 1, 8 (and 15) | Metabolized to intermediates that inhibit DNA or RNA synthesis | 20–30 | Myelosupression, skin rashes, liver transaminitis, allergy, N and V |
| Vinorelbine | 30 mg/m$^2$ day 1 and 8, iv every 3 weeks | Prevent microtubule assembly | 15–25 | Myelosupression, peripheral neuropathy (motor/ sensory autonomic), thrombophlebitis, V |

N and V = nausea and vomiting

Median time to progression and overall survival were significantly longer with docetaxel than MV (19 vs. 11 weeks and 11.4 vs. 8.7 months, respectively).[14] Paclitaxel has also shown to be effective and has shown similar response rates and progression-free survival compared to cyclophosphamide, methotrexate, fluorouracil, and prednisolone (CMFP) (29% and 5.3 months for paclitaxel versus 35% and 6.4 months for CMFP).[15]

Both taxanes can also be given in a weekly schedule, and there is now some evidence suggesting that paclitaxel may be more effective given weekly. The dose-limiting toxicity of paclitaxel is myelosupression and other toxicities include peripheral neuropathy, alopecia, artharalgia, mucositis, and acute hypersensitivity reactions. Adequate premedication with steroids, antihistamine, and H2-receptor antagonists helps to prevent these reactions. Docetaxel cause myelosupression but it is also associated with skin reactions, nail changes, peripheral oedema due to fluid retention, peripheral neuropathy, and hypersensitivity reactions. Careful monitoring and dose modification of taxanes is essential due to its neuropathy as it can adversely affect the quality of life.

## Antimetabolites

**Fluorouracil** Fluorouracil (FU) is one of the antimetabolites that has shown efficacy in metastatic breast cancer. Oral flouropyrimidines capecitabine (Xeloda®) and uftoral (Tegafur®) are rationally designed to generate FU preferentially in tumour tissue and to mimic continuous infusion of FU. The higher concentration of thymidine phosphorylase enzyme in the tumour compared to normal tissue leads to a higher concentration of FU being produced in the tumour. The oral administration of the drug makes it a very popular choice among this cohort of patients where symptom control is the main aim. Capecitabine has been studied extensively and as a monotherapy has shown to produce a 15–26% response and median survival of 1 year in anthracycline and taxane pretreated patients.[16]

Common toxicities seen in these patients include palmar plantar erythema, diarrhoea, nausea, vomiting, and fatigue. It does not cause significant myelosupression or alopecia. The kidney excretes capecitabine metabolites and as a result dose modification is necessary where there is impaired renal function. Mild or moderate hepatic impairment is not an indication for dose reduction but careful monitoring of liver function is important.

**Gemcitabine** Gemcitabine is also an antimetabolite that has shown single-agent activity in metastatic breast cancer. Response rates range between 20 and 30% in phase II trials and commonest toxicities include myelosupression, allergy, rashes, and liver transaminitis.[17]

## Vinca alkaloids

Vinka alkaloids such as Navelbine® act by inhibiting microtubule assembly. It has a reported response rate of 15–25 % in patients pre-treated with taxanes and anthracycline.[18] Main toxicities include myelosupression, peripheral neuropathy, phlebitis, vomiting (Table 1.2). Vinorelbine does not cause alopecia and this is one of the important agents that can be used in women who are reluctant to lose their hair. The neuropathy due to vinorelbine causes loss of motor function, numbness, and autonomic neuropathy leading to constitipation or abdominal cramps.

## Combination chemotherapy

Metastatic breast cancer without prior exposure to anthracycline should have a doxorubicin or epirubicin-containing regimen as first-line treatment. Frequently used, anthracycline-containing regimens include doxorubicin and cyclophosphamide (AC) or fluorouracil, cyclophosphamide, and epirubicin/doxorubicin (FEC or FAC) with response rates of 50–80%.[19] The French epirubicin study group, which compared FEC and FAC, showed that the response rate was 52% and 50%, respectively. Median survivals in the two groups were similar, but the epirubicin-containing combination had a better safety profile. The patients not fit to have an anthracycline-based combination or have underlying comorbidities could have cyclophosphamide, methotrexate, and fluorouracil (CMF). This was one of the first combinations used in metastatic breast cancer.[10]

Docetaxel and capecitabine is one of the most effective doublets and a randomized phase III trial that compared docetaxel and capecitabine with docetaxel alone showed that the combination had a superior response rate (42% vs. 30%), time to disease progression (median 6.1 vs. 4.2 months, p <0.001) and overall survival (14.5 vs. 11.5 months; p = 0.0126).[20] However, there was significant toxicity in the combination treatment arm with 59% and 51% of the patients requiring dose reduction in docetaxel and capecitabine, respectively. Thirty-one per cent of the patients in the combination arm had grade 3 or 4 toxicity, and including grade 2 toxicity this rises to 68%. UK oncologists have used this proven regimen sparingly, despite its efficacy, because of the profound effect of this level of toxicity on quality of life in patients with metastatic disease.

Paclitaxel and gemcitabine is another combination that has shown encouraging activity in metastatic breast cancer. A phase III trial has shown a response rate of 39% with the combination compared with 25% to single agent paclitaxel.[21, 22] The time to progression and overall survival were superior with the combination regimen (5.4 vs. 3.5 months; p = 0.0013). This is a new regimen, which is likely to be more popular with patients and their oncologists because of considerably less side-effects than other regimens (see above).

## Duration of treatment – intermittent or continuous chemotherapy – single agent or combination chemotherapy?

With the development of newer agents prolongation of survival has become a goal in the metastatic setting. Although the long-term survival benefits are modest, many patients are living longer with minimal disease related-symptoms. The decision-making process concerned with which agents to choose is complex and requires tailoring depending on the symptoms, patient fitness, tumour burden, age, and acceptable treatment-related toxicities. An estimation of the overall survival and a gain from the treatment should be discussed in a multidisciplinary setting with the patient. For a small cohort of people, young patients with a good performance status and limited metastatic disease, long-term survival is a possibility and the disease should be managed aggressively according to the wishes of the patient. For the majority of patients with metastatic breast cancer, cure is not a goal of treatment and more conservative treatments with respect to associated toxicities are preferred.

Treatment duration is an important factor that needs to be considered when treating patients in a palliative setting. The benefit of the treatment has to be balanced against the toxicity and its effect on the quality of life. Several studies have compared intermittent with continuous chemotherapy and have shown that although time to treatment failure is longer with continuous treatment, there is no overall survival benefit, although a meta-analysis has shown a survival benefit with longer treatment.[23,24] When quality of life was measured, toxicity from chemotherapy was outweighed by a reduction in disease-related symptoms. There is therefore some evidence to suggest that it is best to continue therapy until disease progression, cessation of clinical benefit, or development of unacceptable toxicities.

## Surgery for metastatic breast cancer

Spinal cord compression due to metastatic bone disease in the vertebral column is a complication of breast cancer, and careful management of cord compression by the oncologists is essential to maintain mobility and to prevent morbidity. Although the standard treatment is steroids and radiotherapy, there is emerging evidence that surgical decompression leads to effective preservation of functional capacities for longer. A randomized study comparing state-of-the-art surgical decompression plus radiotherapy with radiotherapy alone, showed that patients having surgery maintained their mobility for longer and had a higher rate of functional preservation.[25] Therefore, those patients with limited vertebral metastasis without rapidly progressive visceral disease should be considered for spinal decompression surgery with stabilization. There is further discussion of this in Chapter 9.

Patients with rare complications, such as bowel obstruction, may also be managed aggressively depending on the patient's performance status, personal wishes, and the risks and benefits of the procedure.

## Targeted therapy

Targeted therapies are an exciting area in the management of solid malignancies and have many advantages compared to chemotherapy. They are directed at specific molecular targets so are less toxic (e.g. herceptin for human epidermal receptor-2 overexpressing breast cancers, cetuximab for epidermal growth factor-1 over-expressing colonic cancers) and so achieve palliation without affecting the quality of life.

### Herceptin-effective targeted agent

Herceptin (Trastuzumab®) is a monoclonal antibody against the human epidermal receptor-2 (HER-2), which is over-expressed in 25–30% of breast cancers. The majority of HER-2-positive cancers are ER-negative and these patients have more visceral disease; as a result these patients have a poor prognosis with shortened disease-free survival and overall survival. HER-2 is a transmembrane protein with an extracellular ligand-binding domain and an intracellular tyrosine kinase domain, which has a growth regulatory activity. Herceptin binds to HER-2 and inhibits its activity as well as promoting antibody-dependent cell cytotoxicity against the tumour cells. The effect of herceptin is synergistic with cisplatin, carboplatin, and docetaxel while the effect is additive with paclitaxel, doxorubicin, and cyclophoaphamide.

Herceptin is only effective in those breast cancers that over-express HER-2. The pivotal trial involving herceptin and chemotherapy (taxanes or anthracycline) showed that it has a higher response rate, time to disease progression, and a statistically significant survival advantage when these two modalities of treatment are combined.[26] The response rate was 50% with chemotherapy and herceptin while it was 32% with chemotherapy alone. The common toxicities seen with herceptin therapy include fevers, chills (during infusions), and there is a small risk of anaphylactic reactions. The most significant toxicity is the cardiac toxicity that is especially associated with an anthracycline–herceptin combination in the trial and it is not licensed to be combined with an anthracycline.

Patients started on herceptin can be continued on treatment until disease progression even after discontinuation of the chemotherapeutic agents. In fact there is *in vitro* data to suggest that herceptin is effective as long as it is around and withdrawal of herceptin could lead to rapid tumour growth. Another chemotherapeutic agent could be introduced as the disease progresses while on herceptin.

## Case studies

### Case 1

A 43-year-old lady had a mastectomy in 1994 but was diagnosed with liver metastasis postoperatively. The tumour was ER-positive and the patient had FAC chemotherapy. In 1995, she received high-dose chemotherapy and a bone marrow transplant in Australia. In 1996, the carcinoembryonic antigen (CEA) was climbing and a scan showed a solitary liver metastasis, which was surgically resected and she was started on tamoxifen. She subsequently relapsed in the liver, in 1997, was started on CMF with prednisolone, and had a good partial response. She was started on megace at the end of treatment in 1998. In 1999, the liver metastases progressed again and endocrine therapy was changed to anastrazole. When she progressed again she was started on docetaxel and, as she was HER-2 negative, herceptin was not given. She had six cycles and had neurotoxicity and nail toxicity. She was started on exemestane at the end of taxanes and was rechallenged with epirubicin for four cycles when her liver metastases progressed but there was no response to this treatment. The patient was started on maintenance tamoxifen. Her liver metastases progressed in the middle of 2001 and she was started on oral capecitabine; she had this for a total of 2 years. She had a very good response and her quality of life was maintained. Unfortunately, by the end of 2 years she started getting severe palmar plantar erythema and diarrhoea. Her liver metastases progressed as well and she was commenced on vinorelbine and carboplatin. She had severe autonomic neuropathy due to vinorelbine and thrombocytopenia due to carboplatin. There was no response to treatment as well. She was started on gemcitabine at this point but became too unwell and she was transferred to a hospice for her final days. She had good palliation of symptoms and a quality of life with the treatment and survived 10 years with a liver metastasis.

## Case 2

A 43-year-old lady had a mastectomy and axillary clearance for a 23 mm grade 1 infiltrating ductal carcinoma in 1996. She also suffers from insulin dependent diabetes mellitus and polymyalgia rheumatica. She is a pharmacist with two teenage children. Postoperatively she was treated with radiotherapy and tamoxifen. She presented in March 2002 with neck pain and a 'tingling feeling' in the hand. A neck X-ray showed bony destruction at C7 vertebra for which she had radiotherapy and was started on Zoladex. In August 2002, she was admitted with nausea, vomiting, and upper abdominal pain. At this admission she was anaemic and had hypercalcaemia. A further bone scan showed progressive disease with new areas of disease only in the bone. The blood picture was highly suggestive of marrow infiltration and this was confirmed by a bone marrow biopsy. The liver function tests and renal function were abnormal as well. She was started on weekly epirubicin chemotherapy because of the multiple organ dysfunction. Three-weekly pamidronate was also started because of the symptomatic bone metastasis. She was initially dependent on regular transfusions to maintain the haemoglobin but as the time progressed the blood count improved and she became less dependent on transfusions. When the blood counts recovered she was started on three-weekly epirubicin. She had a few delays in treatment because of low blood counts but no other significant toxicity. Following completion of chemotherapy she was started on anastrazole. The restaging investigations showed that the bone metastasis have improved with chemotherapy. Sixteen months later, she developed some pelvic pain and a bone scan showed progressive disease following which she had radiotherapy to the pubic rami and her aromatase inhibitor was changed to exemestane. She also started to get headaches from the skull vault metastasis which were treated with radiotherapy. When she was restaged she still had stable bone disease and continues on endocrine therapy. This lady has maintained a very good quality of life even though she has had metastatic breast cancer for over two years.

## References

1 Peto, R., Boreham, J., Clarke, M. *et al.* (2000). UK and USA breast cancer deaths down 25% in year 2000 at ages 20–69 years. *Lancet*, 355, 1822.

2 Chia, S.K.L., Speers, C., Kang, A., *et al.* (2003). The impact of new chemotherapeutic and hormonal agents on the survival of women with metastatic breast cancer (MBC) in a population cohort. *Pro Am Soc Clin Oncol*, 22, 6, Abstract 22.

3 Giordano, S., Buzdar, A.U., Kau, S.C., and Hortobagyi, G.N. (2002). Improvements in breast cancer survival: results from MD Anderson Cancer Centre protocols from 1975–2000. *Pro Am Soc Clin Oncol*, 21, 30, Abstract 212.

4 Beatson, G.Y. (1896). On the treatment of inoperable cases of carcinoma of the mamma: suggestions for a new method of treatment, with illustrative cases. *Lancet*, 2, 104–107.

5 Mourisden, H., Gershanovich, M., Sun, Y., *et al.* (2003). Phase III study of letrozole versus tamoxifen as first-line therapy of advanced breast cancer in post-menopausal women: Analysis of survival and update of efficacy from the International Letrozole Breast Cancer Group. *J Clin Oncol*, 21, 2101–2109.

6 Bonneterre, J., Thurlimann, B., Robertson, J.F.R., *et al.* (2000). Anastrazole versus tamoxifen as first-line therapy for advanced breast cancer in 668 post-menopausal women: Results

of the tamoxifen and arimidex randomised group efficacy and tolerability study. *J Clin Oncol*, 18, 3748–3757.

7 Kaufmann, M., Bajetta, E., Dirix, L.Y. *et al.* (2000). Exemestane is superior to megestrol acetate after tamoxifen failure in post-menopausal women with advanced breast cancer: results of a phase III randomised double-blind trial. The Exemestane Study Group. *J Clin Oncol*, 11,1399–1411.

8 Howells, A., Robertson, J.F.R., Albano, Q.J., *et al.* (2002). Fulvestrant, formerly ICI 182,780, Is as effective as anastrazole in postmenopausal women with advanced breast cancer progressing after prior endocrine treatment. *J Clin Oncol*, 20, 3396–3403.

9 Klijn, J.G.M., Blamey, R.W., Boccardo, F., *et al.* (2001). Combined tamoxifen and luteinising hormonal-releasing hormone (LHRH) agonist or LHRH agonist alone in premenopausal advanced breast cancer: A meta-analysis of four randomised trials. *J Clin Oncol*, 19, 343–353.

10 Ellis, M.J., Coop, A., Singh, B., *et al.* (2001). Letrozole is more effective neoadjuvant endocrine therapy than tamoxifen for ErbB-1- and/or Erb-2 positive, oestrogen receptor positive primary breast cancer: evidence from a phase III randomised trial. *J Clin Oncol*, 19, 3808–3816.

11 Fossati, R., Confalonieri, C., Torri, V., *et al.* (1998). Cytotoxic and hormonal treatment for metastatic breast cancer: A systemic review of published randomised trials involving 31510 women. *J Clin Oncol*, 16, 3439–3460.

12 French Epirubicin Study Group (1998). A prospective randomised phase III trial comparing combination chemotherapy with cyclophosphamide, fluorouracil, and either doxorubicin or epirubicin. *J Clin Oncol*, 6, 679–688.

13 Earl, H. and Iddawela, M. (2004). Epirubicin as adjuvant treatment in breast cancer. *Expert Rev Anticancer Ther*, 4, 89–95.

14 Nabholtz, J.M., Senn, H.J., Bezwoda, W.R., *et al.* (1999). Prospective randomised trial of docetaxel versus mitomycin plus vinblastine in patients with metastatic breast cancer progressing despite previous chemotherapy-chemotherapy. *J Clin Oncol*, 17, 1314–1324.

15 Bishop, J.F., Dewer, J., Toner, G.C., *et al.* (1999). Initial paclitaxel improves outcome compared with CMFP combination chemotherapy as front-line therapy in untreated metastatic breast cancer. *J Clin Oncol*, 17, 2355–2364.

16 Esteva, F.J., Valero, V., Puszatai, L., *et al.* (2001). Chemotherapy of metastatic breast cancer: what to expect in 2001 and beyond. *Oncologist*, 6, 133–146.

17 Yardley, D.A. (2004). Gemcitabine and docetaxel in metastatic and neoadjuvant treatment of breast cancer. *Semin Oncol*, 31, 37–44.

18 Venturino, A., Comandini, D., Simoni, C., *et al.* (2000). Is salvage chemotherapy for metastatic breast cancer always effective and well tolerated? A phase II randomised trail of vinorelbine versus 5-flourouracil plus leucovorin versus combination of mitoxantrone, 5-rlourouracil plus leucovorin. *Breast Cancer Res Treat*, 60, 195–200.

19 Nabholtz, J.M., Reese, D.M., Lindsay, M.A., and Riva, A. (2002). Combination chemotherapy for metastatic breast cancer. *Expert Rev Anticancer Ther*, 2, 169–180.

20 O'Shaughnessy, J., Miles, D., Vukelja, S., *et al.* (2002). Superior survival with capecitabine plus docetaxel combination in anthracycline-pretreated patients with advanced breast cancer: Phase III trail result. *J Clin Oncol*, 12, 2812–2823.

21 O'Shaughnessy, J., Nag, S., Calderillo-Ruis, G., *et al.* (2003). Gemcitabine and paclitaxel versus paclitaxel as first-line treatment for anthracycline pre-treated metastatic breast cancer (MBC): Interim results of a global phase III study. *Pro Am Soc Clin Oncol*, 22, 7, 25.

22  Albain, K.S., Nag, S., Calderillo-Ruiz, G., *et al.* (2004). Global phase III study of gemcitabine plus paclitaxel (GT) vs. paclitaxel as frontline therapy for metastatic breast cancer: First report of overall survival. *Pro Am Soc Clin Oncol*, **23**, 5, 510.

23  Muss, H.B., Case, L.D., Richards, F., *et al.* (1991). Interrupted versus continuous chemotherapy in patients with metastatic breast cancer. *N Engl J Med*, **325**, 1342–1348.

24  Coates, A.S., Stockler, M., and Wilcken, N. (2003). Controversies in metastatic breast cancer: optimal duration of chemotherapy. In: Perry MC, ed. American Society of Clinical Oncology Education Book. **39**, 119–121. American Society of Clinical Oncology, Alexandria, VA.

25  Patchell, R., Tibbs, P.A., Regine, W.F., *et al* (2003). A randomised trial of direct decompressive surgical resection of spinal cord compression by metastasis. *Proc Am Soc Clin Oncol*, **22**, 1.

26  Slamon, D.J., Leyland-Jones, B., Shak, S., *et al.* (2001). Use of chemotherapy plus monoclonal antibody against HER-2 for metastatic breast cancer that over expresses HER-2. *N Engl J Med* **344**, 783–792.

Chapter 2

# Pain control in advanced local disease

Angela Bentley and Marie Fallon

## Summary

This chapter addresses the causes, assessment, and management of pain in advanced local breast cancer. Using the WHO analgesic ladder as the basis for cancer pain management, we also describe other methods (pharmacological and non-pharmacological) of pain control that can be used in specific pain syndromes in patients with advanced local disease.

## Sources of evidence

We have stated, where possible, the type of evidence that is available for the use of the strategies we discuss. There are few randomized, controlled trials in this area of palliative medicine, and evidence for the use of some drugs comes from non-malignant pain trials, particularly in neuropathic pain. Case reports have been used, if trials have not been available. In areas where evidence is sparse we have used 'accepted practice' from leading palliative care authors and our own clinical experience.

## Definition

Advanced local breast disease can be the first presentation of the disease, or can be due to local recurrence of a previously treated breast cancer. In those presenting with a primary tumour the term 'locally advanced breast cancer' is commonly used. There is some variation in definition but ordinarily, using the TNM classification, includes T3 or T4 tumours or N2, N3 tumours of any size (Table 2.1). In developed countries, depending on clinical definitions, between 5 and 10% of patients with breast cancer can present with locally advanced disease. These cancers are biologically heterogeneous and range from slow-growing, sometimes neglected, cancers to the very aggressive. Inflammatory breast cancer is rare and characterized by indurated, oedematous and erythematous skin changes, and has a poorer prognosis. Local recurrence can arise in the treated breast or chest wall or axilla. The clinical diversity of advanced local breast disease is matched by the variety of causes of pain in this group of patients.

## Assessment

### Getting started

Before embarking on the assessment of pain it is useful to have an understanding of the different causes of pain associated with advanced local breast cancer, remembering that several factors can coexist.

### Skin involvement

Malignant infiltration of the skin and its supporting blood and lymphatic vessels is common in advanced local disease, resulting in painful skin nodules or fungating or ulcerating malignant wounds. Bacterial infection often coexists, causing an exudate and malodour. In inflammatory cancers diffuse infiltration of the skin can be clinically difficult to distinguish from cellulitis. Relentless, progressive spread of cancer cells in the dermis and dermal lymphatics, leading to extensive infiltration and eventual fibrosis of the chest wall, is characteristic of carcinoma 'en cuirasse'. Damaged or ulcerated skin, bacterial infection, and wound exudates produce local inflammation and pain. If tumour infiltration causes cutaneous nerve compression neuropathic pain can result.

Up to 20% of patients develop a postmastectomy pain syndrome following breast cancer surgery.[1] This is a neuropathic pain syndrome, usually attributed to injury of the intercostobrachial nerve; it is characterized by abnormal sensation in the axilla and medial aspect of the arm. It does not signify recurrent disease but needs to be distinguished from pain caused by local recurrence.

### Chest wall

Given the close proximity of the chest wall to the breast it is not surprising that, in advanced local disease, musculoskeletal pain can occur if the tumour becomes fixed to underlying muscle (intercostal, serratus anterior). Further local progression can lead to rib erosion. Pain can arise from direct bone involvement, with tenderness over the area of erosion, or from intercostal nerve damage producing radicular, unilateral neuropathic pain in the distribution of the compressed nerve.

### Brachial plexus

In advanced local disease damage to the brachial plexus can be a consequence of various factors: tumour infiltration by axillary nodes or supraclavicular fossa nodes, thrombus formation, postradiation fibrosis, or lymphoedema. The pain is characteristically neuropathic, with numbness, allodynia, paraesthesia, and hyperaesthesia. In the majority of cases caused by breast cancer, the lower plexus (C7–T1) is involved, with pain in the shoulder radiating to the elbow, medial aspect of the forearm, and into the 4th and 5th fingers. The upper plexus (C5, C6) is more commonly affected by supraclavicular nodal disease or in postradiation fibrosis, and pain is often distributed along the shoulder girdle, biceps, ulnar aspect of the forearm, and into the thumb and index finger.

Sympathetically maintained pain or complex regional pain syndrome is rare but can occur if tumour infiltration involves the sympathetic chain. Allodynia and focal autonomic dysregulation (sweating, vasomotor, or trophic changes) are key features.

The distribution of the pain is related to the pattern of vascular innervation rather than to the dermatomal pattern of the peripheral nerves.

## Lymphoedema

Between 25 and 28% of patients treated for breast cancer develop upper limb lymphoedema.[2] Axillary surgery and radiotherapy disrupts the deep lymphatic system of the arm resulting in tissue swelling. Tumour recurrence in the axilla and further damage to the lymphatic system by dermal and subcutaneous infiltration can exacerbate the situation causing intractable lymphoedema. Lymphoedema may be a presenting feature in those with an advanced primary tumour.

Clinically, lymphoedema can range from mild, asymptomatic swelling to a grossly swollen, deformed and dysfunctional arm. Although lymphoedema is not commonly regarded as an essentially painful process, about a quarter of patients report significant pain.[3]

Several types of pain associated with upper limb lymphoedema have been described.[4] The weight of the arm can aggravate inflammatory arthropathies (e.g. arthritis, bursitis, tendonitis) and cause myofascial pain, characterized by muscle spasm, shoulder joint stiffness, and limitation of movement. Arm swelling can cause entrapment neuropathies, most commonly carpal tunnel syndrome, though rarely a brachial plexopathy. Pain can increase acutely in the presence of thrombophlebitis or deep vein thrombosis. The management of lymphoedema is discussed further in Chapter 5.

## History

The start of good pain management begins with a thorough pain assessment. It should allow a clinical hypothesis about the cause or causes of the pain to be made, which will then guide decision-making about the types of therapeutic interventions which may be beneficial.

The context in which the pain is occurring is important. Patients should be sensitively asked about the background history to their disease and any previous treatment. Advanced local disease is sometimes the result of a deliberately or subconsciously concealed carcinoma-usually in an elderly woman, though occasionally it may happen in the younger age groups. Particular sensitivity is needed in these cases because although a minority are quite clear-eyed about what they have done (avoiding treatment at an advanced age )some are wracked with guilt and self-blame, once the disease is diagnosed, at not presenting earlier. The families, partners and friends often have mixed emotions-they feel excluded and sometimes very angry at their relative for 'keeping them out', particularly when it becomes clear that the cancer could have been easily and atraumatically treated by endocrine therapy alone.

When evaluating pain the basics are important. It is necessary to ask about the site, quality (e.g. burning sensation, dull ache) and intensity of the pain. The temporal pattern and the circumstances surrounding the onset of the pain need to be clarified. Factors that relieve or exacerbate the pain ought to be noted. Changes in temperature can affect neuropathic pain, and heat can increase lymphoedema leading to worsening pain. It is useful to ask about any associated symptoms or signs (e.g. pyrexia and erythema in cellulitis, altered sensation and motor weakness in neuropathic pain). The impact that pain has on the activities of daily living, and on the patient's emotional and social well-being, should be explored with delicacy. It can also be beneficial to find out a patient's own understanding about the meaning of the pain, and what it signifies to them. Discovering the patient's response to current or previous analgesia and non-pharmacological therapies can assist further management.

## Examination

Medical and neurological examination is valuable in the clinical assessment of pain. Any examination should be performed sensitively, particularly in patients with advanced local breast disease who may be self-conscious about their body image or the presence of malodorous wounds. Clearly, performing a rigorous examination on a very frail patient close to the end of life may be inappropriate, especially if it will not alter the pain management.

Knowledge of particular cancer pain syndromes (e.g. brachial plexopathy) and the patient's history can guide the examination. Initial general observations of the patient can be informative about the effect that pain is having on physical functioning (e.g. unable to move arm due to pain) and emotional well-being (e.g. withdrawn or tearful patient).

On examination, there may be surgical scars or stigmata of radiotherapy treatment. The site of pain ought to be visually inspected and palpated to elicit areas of tenderness. In myofascial pain muscular 'trigger points' that reproduce pain on palpation are found.[5] Any skin changes or other physical signs (e.g. palpable axillary nodes) should be noted. A neurological examination assessing motor and sensory changes can help define any neurological damage. Sensory abnormalities might include allodynia, hyperaesthesia, and alteration in thermal sensation. It can be useful to examine the impact of physical changes on functional ability to highlight activities of daily living that may require assistance.

## Investigations

As noted previously the context in which the pain is occurring is important and investigations can be used to identify the site and extent of the tumour. Whether advanced local disease is the primary presentation or represents local relapse, the diagnosis is usually confirmed histologically and formal staging investigations are undertaken.

Investigations can help confirm our clinical suspicions as to the aetiology of the pain. Whilst routine blood tests may not inform our understanding of the possible cause(s) of the pain they can help direct our choice of analgesia (e.g. avoiding non-steroidal anti-inflammatory drugs in those with renal impairment). Plain X-rays or a bone scan can be useful in suspected rib erosion. A computed tomography (CT) scan of the thorax can assess tumour infiltration into chest wall musculature. Both CT and magnetic resonance imaging (MRI) scanning can demonstrate characteristic features of lymphoedema and may also be valuable in excluding or confirming a malignant cause of lymphoedema. MRI is sensitive for brachial plexus lesions, and there is some work investigating the combination of MRI scanning with position emission tomography (PET) scanning for recurrent local breast cancer.[6]

A negative radiological investigation does not necessarily rule out a malignant cause for the pain and it should be reviewed with the radiologist to compare radiological findings with the clinical picture. It has been shown that pain from malignant brachial plexus lesions can *precede* neurological and radiological findings by several weeks or months.[7] In these circumstances a pragmatic approach is usually adopted where pain control is optimized and investigations are repeated if pain worsens or physical or neurological signs develop. Obviously, this can be a difficult situation for the patient and they may require additional support to cope with the uncertainty.

Whilst investigations can help our knowledge about the disease status it is important to ensure that we do not burden patients with very advanced debilitating disease with unnecessary tests, the results of which would not alter the management of their pain.

## Who else may be of help

Patients with advanced local breast cancer need to be managed by a multidisciplinary team rather than by a practitioner working in isolation. The professional skills needed to give each patient the best treatment will very much depend on the patient's particular circumstances.

It can be helpful to discuss with a breast surgeon or oncologist whether surgery or cancer treatment could benefit tumour-related pain. The advice of an anaesthetist specializing in pain management will be needed if invasive procedures such as nerve blocks are being considered. Review and discussion of radiology investigations with a radiologist can be useful clinically. Clinical psychologists can help with specific psychological pain control techniques or if anxiety or depression are present. Physiotherapy and occupational therapy should be available to facilitate maintenance of function and independence. Access to skilled wound care is vitally important to those with fungating or ulcerating malignant lesions. Patients and their families often benefit from the support of a breast cancer clinical nurse specialist or clinical nurse specialist in palliative care.

Hospice services, such as community palliative care teams and day hospice, can provide useful symptom control and psychosocial support for patients and relatives. When pain is an ongoing problem, inpatient hospice care may be appropriate for pain management.

## Management

### General pain management

Following the assessment it is important to consider whether a primary therapy (i.e. treatment that addresses the underlying cause of the pain) could help the pain. A course of antibiotics may help pain from cellulitis. Pain from tumour infiltration may benefit from antitumour treatment, such as surgery, radiotherapy, chemotherapy, or hormonal manipulation. Even if a potentially reversible cause of pain is found, it is common that specific analgesic treatments are also needed.

Analgesia should be given regularly and with the availability of an appropriate breakthrough analgesia.[8] The World Health Organization (WHO) Three Step Analgesic Ladder provides a useful method for drug selection in cancer pain, using the conventional classification of analgesic drugs – non-opioids, opioids, and adjuvants.[9] The WHO 'analgesic ladder' was not designed to be used in isolation and other

**Table 2.1** TNM classification of breast cancer

| Stage | Definition |
|-------|------------|
| T3 | Tumour more than 5 cm |
| T4a | Tumour extending into the chest wall |
| T4b | Oedema, including peau d'orange, or ulceration of the breast skin or satellite nodules confined to the same breast |
| T4c | Both T4a and b |
| T4d | Inflammatory carcinoma<br>Diffuse brawny infiltration of the skin, often no underlying mass |
| N2 | Fixed axillary nodes |
| N3 | Ipsilateral internal mammary lymph node metastases |

strategies, which are discussed below, are often required, particularly in patients with advanced local breast cancer.

The principles guiding the use of the analgesic ladder are that:

1 selection of analgesia is dependent on the severity of the pain rather than the stage of the disease;
2 if pain is not controlled at one step then there should be a move up to the next step;
3 adjuvant drugs should be used when necessary at any of the steps and selection is dependent on the pathophysiology of the pain;
4 it is also important to anticipate and treat the common side-effects of analgesic medication (e.g. nausea, constipation).

## Non-opioids

Paracetamol is a useful analgesic for mild-to-moderate pain, and is often combined with a weak opioid as a single preparation at Step 2 (e.g. cocodamol).

Non-steroidal anti-inflammatory drugs have a vital role in most forms of cancer pain, particularly those pains associated with inflammation. Common side-effects include gastrointestinal toxicity, fluid retention, and renal failure. Newer agents, known as COX-2 inhibitors, appear to have less gastrotoxic effects but may be more prothrombotic.[10] A review of the cardiovascular and cerebrovascular safety of all COX-2 drugs is currently underway but rofecoxib (Vioxx) has recently been withdrawn by MERCK because of emerging data from the APPROVe trial that patients taking this drug for over 18 months had an increased risk of cardiovascular events compared to placebo. Celecoxib is in a different class from rofecoxib and the former may be safer. Further data are awaited. Any risk has to be weighed against the benefits in a patient with a life-limiting illness and a painful complication.

The 'ceiling' effect of analgesia in the non-opioids limits dose escalation.

## Opioids

Opioids are excellent analgesics. The starting dose and rate of titration will vary between individuals. Whilst there is no pharmacological ceiling dose for opioids, in practice dose escalation is limited by unacceptable side-effects. Gastrointestinal side-effects are common and should be anticipated. Central nervous system side-effects are generally dose related. Persistent sedation, confusion, hallucinations, and myoclonus suggest that a 'ceiling' dose has been reached.

In circumstances where pain is controlled, a gradual decrease in opioid dose may be possible. If pain continues, employing other methods of managing pain (e.g. other adjuvant drugs, primary therapy, non-pharmacological strategies) can reduce opioid requirements. From pharmacogenomic work it is known that individuals respond differently to the various opioids,[11] so for patients who develop intolerable side-effects but who have opioid-responsive pain switching opioid can often be beneficial.[12] In clinical practice this is often oxycodone or fentanyl in the first instance, with a switch to methadone being used as second line, or in cases where pain control is clearly difficult.

Methadone in addition to being an opioid receptor agonist may be an NMDA (N-methyl-D-aspartate) receptor blocker. Methadone has been shown to be helpful and well tolerated in some patients who have a poor analgesic response and unacceptable side-effects with morphine.[13] There are large interindividual variations in the equianalgesic ratio of methadone to other opioids.[14] It interacts with a number of drugs and also has a long and variable half-life, which can lead to accumulation and adverse effects. Specialist supervision of its use is recommended.

## Adjuvant analgesia

This is a term for a heterogeneous collection of drugs which have analgesic properties in some conditions, including anticonvulsants (e.g. gabapentin), antidepressants (e.g. amitriptyline), corticosteroids (e.g. dexamethasone), and N-methyl-D-aspartate (NMDA) receptor channel blockers (e.g. ketamine).[15] By acting in a different way to opioids, adjuvant analgesia can be useful in providing a better balance between pain control and side-effects, and is of particular importance in the management of neuropathic pain. The selection of the drug is dependent on the pathophysiology of the pain, but some of the other properties of the drug may be utilized in an effort to manage other symptoms (e.g. amitriptyline used for neuropathic pain may concurrently improve low mood).

## Invasive anaesthetic techniques

In some patients, despite the use of systemic medication, pain control may remain inadequate. The use of interventional anaesthetic pain techniques has been called the '4th Step' on the WHO analgesic ladder and there are circumstances where these can be helpful in advanced local disease.[5] Before embarking on invasive procedures it is important that other strategies, including non-pharmacological and psychosocial approaches, have also been considered.

# Pain control for specific syndromes

The WHO analgesic ladder forms the basis to cancer pain management, but these drugs are often usefully complemented by others to obtain a better balance between pain control and side-effects.

## Pain from skin involvement

Topical analgesia that has little systemic absorption has the potential advantage of reducing or avoiding the use of conventional medications and their associated side-effects.

Topical local anaesthetics such as EMLA (lidocaine 2.5%, prilocaine 2.5%) and lidocaine gel can be helpful in the treatment of painful cutaneous nodules and malignant ulcerating lesions, though the evidence, so far, is anecdotal.[16]

Evidence that opioid receptors are detectable in peripheral nerve terminals in the presence of inflammation has led to topical opioid usage.[17] Two small, randomized, controlled studies have shown that diamorphine and morphine gels produce local analgesia without systemic adverse effects in painful pressure ulcers.[18,19] Anecdotal evidence exists for its effectiveness in ulcerated lesions secondary to breast cancer.[20] Further work is required to investigate the optimal dose strength and frequency. It is our clinical practice to mix 5–10 mg of diamorphine, dissolved in 0.1 ml of water for injection, with 15 mg of intrasite gel. This is applied to the wound usually on a daily basis. Patients may need anything from once daily up to four times daily application.

Topical capsaicin cream has been shown to be effective in postmastectomy pain in cancer patients.[21] As capsaicin can initially cause a poorly tolerated, local burning sensation during the first 2–3 days of application of capsaicin, the cream should be preceded by local anaesthetic cream to prevent an unpleasant burning sensation.

## Pain from chest wall involvement

A local anaesthetic intercostal nerve block is a very effective method of controlling pain from an eroded rib.[22] Intrapleural local anaesthetics have been shown to be effective in producing multiple unilateral intercostal nerve blocks, and can be useful for chest wall and rib disease.[23]

## Neuropathic brachial plexus pain

Although neuropathic pain is often considered to be poorly responsive to opioid therapy there is no evidence to suggest that it is truly 'opioid-resistant'. The first-line approach to treatment of moderate to severe neuropathic pain should be opioid therapy. Adjuvant therapy should normally be considered at the same time as starting standard analgesic therapy.

### Adjuvant analgesia

Although there are no controlled trials evaluating antidepressants or anticonvulsants in cancer-related neuropathic pain, conventional practice supports their early use based on controlled trials in a variety of neuropathic pain syndromes.[24]

Tricyclic antidepressants (e.g. amitriptyline), selective serotonin reuptake inhibitors (e.g. citalopram), noradrenaline selective serotonin reuptake inhibitors (e.g. venlafaxine) are used. The evidence is significantly stronger for tricyclic antidepressants than for the others. Doses need to be titrated carefully until an effective dose is achieved. It can take days to several weeks to achieve the maximum analgesic effect.

Gabapentin is increasingly recommended as the first-line anticonvulsant because it has proven analgesic properties, is well tolerated, and has less drug interactions than other anticonvulsants.[25] Titration needs to be slower for older patients and those with multiple medical problems. Pregabalin offers the potential for easier titration because of target dose tablet size and 12-hourly dosing regimen. There is evidence that it is a more potent analgesic than gabapentin and in some patients who have unacceptable side-effects with gabapentin it can be better tolerated. We start at 75 mg/day and titrate to 300 mg bd.

Corticosteroids have been shown to be of benefit in the treatment of neuropathic pain from infiltration or compression of neural structures and can be helpful in brachial plexopathy pain.[26] The mechanism of action is unclear. In a simplistic way, it may be related to reduction in tumour-associated oedema, however more complex neuropharmacological mechanisms are suspected. There are short and long-term adverse effects related to dose and duration of therapy. Risks of long-term use have to be balanced against the potential benefits.

### N-methyl-D-aspartate (NMDA) receptor blockers

The NMDA receptor is present in the central nervous system and is involved in the 'wind-up' phenomenon associated with neuropathic pain, where central neurones become sensitized following nerve injury. The general anaesthetic agent, ketamine, an NMDA antagonist has undergone extensive investigation recently. Case reports and one small randomized controlled trial have shown its effectiveness in neuropathic cancer pain.[27–29] It is now considered an option in those with severe neuropathic pain, in whom conventional approaches have failed. Adverse effects include dysphoria, delirium, hallucinations, and nightmares but the use of subanaesthetic analgesic doses, and haloperidol or diazepam, reduces the risk of these developing.[29] In the future, NMDA subtype antagonists are likely to be more clinically useful.

### Local anaesthetics

Although oral and intravenous infusions of local anaesthetics have been shown to be effective in randomized controlled trials of neuropathic pain syndromes this has not been replicated in neuropathic cancer pain studies.[30, 31] Their action is due to a reduction in nerve membrane excitability. Anecdotally, long-term subcutaneous lidocaine has been used effectively to control intractable neuropathic cancer pain,[32] and flecainide (oral) has been helpful in pain due to tumour infiltration in cancer patients.[33] In clinical practice, mexiletine is used in preference to flecainide as the risk of serious toxicity is less, and intravenous infusions of lidocaine are used where rapid control of severe neuropathic pain is needed.[34] Adverse effects include dizziness, paraesthesia, tremor, seizures, and cardiac arrhythmias.

### Topical analgesics

The development of a 5% lidocaine patch has made the use of topical analgesics easier. Studies have shown its usefulness in reducing pain and allodynia in a variety of neuropathic pain conditions,[35–37] though cancer-related neuropathic pain has not been specifically addressed. Its tolerability and lack of systemic side-effects make it an attractive option for patients who develop adverse side-effects from the commonly prescribed medication for neuropathic pain.

### Regional blockade

Regional blockade of the brachial plexus can be beneficial in cancer pain.[38] The value of a continuous infusion of local anaesthetic via a catheter placed at the brachial plexus has been demonstrated in intractable neuropathic cancer pain, and techniques are being developed to reduce the risk of catheter-related complications.[39] Neurolytic blockade is usually reserved for patients with a poor prognosis in whom the risk of developing postneurolysis pain is low.[5]

Interpleural analgesia, where local anaesthetic is injected into the pleural space, has been used for brachial plexus and chest wall pain in cancer patients.[23] Continuous or bolus infusions can be given via tunnelled catheters.[40]

Percutaneous cervical cordotomy disrupts the spinothalamic tract. It is now used rarely for intractable unilateral upper limb cancer pain given its permanence and that its complications include sleep apnoea, respiratory dysfunction, and postcordotomy dysaesthetic syndromes.[41]

In sympathetically mediated pain, now known as complex regional pain syndrome, a trial of local anaesthetic sympathetic blockade can be useful.[42] Neurolysis of the stellate ganglion is not usually performed, given its location and the risks of damage to vascular and neurological structures, but repeated local anaesthetic blocks can provide good relief for some patients.[5]

Brachial plexus block may be appropriate for brachial plexus infiltration, axillary block is most effective for analgesia distal to the elbow. Implanted systems to allow continuous infusion of analgesic agents can be effective, however expertise in placement and fixation is very important.

## Lymphoedema-related pain

Massage, relaxation acupuncture, and local anaesthetic injection of trigger points are useful in myofascial pain, though it should be remembered that acupuncture should not be used on a lymphoedematous arm due to the risk of cellulitis.[43,44,5] Muscle relaxants (e.g. diazepam, baclofen) are helpful for muscle spasm. Inflammatory arthropathies are often treated with non-steroidal anti-inflammatory drugs, or local infiltration of steroids followed by physiotherapy. The use of long-term antibiotic prophylaxis can be helpful in recurrent thrombophlebitis.

# Non-pharmacological approaches

It is rare that non-pharmacological approaches alone are sufficient to combat cancer pain, but they have a vital role in complementing drug therapies, and may reduce drug usage and systemic side-effects.

## Physiotherapy

This is a crucial aspect of pain management for patients with advanced local disease. Many physiotherapists are trained in the use of TENS (transcutaneous electrical nerve stimulation), acupuncture, and relaxation techniques that can be so helpful.[45] Correct support and positioning of painful areas is valuable (e.g. cushion supporting a lymphoedematous arm).[43] Low compression garments may minimize increases in lymphoedematous swelling. In ambulant patients with gross arm lymphoedema and weakness from brachial plexus damage a sling can redistribute the weight of the arm.[46] This may improve comfort, balance, and mobility. Gentle exercise can help prevent pain and stiffness in bed-bound patients and help maintain function in mobile patients, but clearly individual circumstances need to be taken into account.[46]

Pain, muscle weakness, and swelling can all interfere with functional ability. An occupational therapist can advise on the use of appliances, adaptations, and retraining in maintaining some independence in activities of daily living.[47]

TENS is thought to work by electrical stimulation of certain nerve fibres blocking signals carrying pain impulses to the brain. There is anecdotal evidence to support the use of TENS for cancer pain and those who respond to TENS gain relief without systemic side-effects.[48] Patients who have difficulty tolerating conventional therapy may therefore benefit from a trial of TENS. It has been shown to reduce lymphoedema and associated pain.

A retrospective audit supports the use of acupuncture for the treatment of pain, particularly muscular spasm and postsurgical syndromes in cancer patients.[44] Acupuncture has also been shown to improve depression in breast cancer patients with pain.[49] To reduce the risk of complications a physician with knowledge of the clinical condition should perform acupuncture.[50]

## Complementary therapies

Although evidence for the use of complementary therapies is scant, some patients will find these methods helpful in controlling their pain, and aromatherapy, the use of plant-based essential oils, can be useful in the presence of malodorous wounds.

## Psychological concerns

Women with breast cancer have been shown to have a high risk of developing psychological difficulties, particularly anxiety and depression. (This is discussed in some depth in Chapter 3.) Pain, lymphoedema, and body image problems are thought to be factors that contribute. Frustration from a loss of independence can add to the emotional distress.[51] Pain signifying tumour progression, can be associated with fear and a sense of hopelessness which then exacerbates the pain and suffering.[52] In general, patients cope better if they feel that their doctor has tried to elicit, understand, and help them with their individual concerns.[51]

Specific psychological interventions can be useful to help the patient cope with the pain. Cognitive–behavioural techniques, such as relaxation, visual imagery or distraction, and hypnosis, have been successfully employed.[53]

## Important palliative care points

Pain can be difficult to control in local advanced breast cancer, and often coexists with very visible signs and symptoms of tumour activity. Alterations in body image, loss of functional ability, and the presence of malodorous wounds can lead to social isolation.

Whilst some patients may wish to continue with work to gain a sense of control and normality, adaptations may be required to their daily routine and environment.[54] For others work may be neither desirable or possible, and the family income may be significantly reduced which causes problems of its own.

Patients and their families both require support, though their needs are often quite different. Given the genetic factors involved in breast cancer the daughters of patients can feel particularly vulnerable. They often provide a care-giving role to their mothers, whilst having to cope with the uncertainty of developing breast cancer themselves. They can also feel that their information and support needs are not well met.[55] Patients can feel anxious and guilty about passing the risk of breast cancer to their daughters.[51] This can all impact on family dynamics. It is important as we strive to control pain that we do not forget the 'person' in the patient.

As with all aspects of cancer care, building a relationship with the patient and her family is the keystone to exploring all aspects of care. Many patients and their families benefit enormously from the comprehensive, multidisciplinary support offered by hospices and specialist palliative care teams. This care should be complementary to that provided by the oncology team and not seen as an alternative.

## References

1 Smith, W.C.S., Bourne, D., Squair, J., Phillips, D.O., and Chambers, W.A. (1999). A retrospective cohort study of post mastectomy pain syndrome. *Pain*, 83, 91–95.

2 Logan, V. (1995). Incidence and prevalence of lymphoedema: a literature review. *J Clin Nurs*, 4, 213–219.

3 Passik, S.D., Newman, M., Brennan, M.J., and Tunkel, R. (1995). Predictors of psychological distress, sexual dysfunction and physical functioning among women with upper extremity lymphoedema related to breast cancer. *Psycho-Oncol*, 4, 255–263.

4 Newman, M., Brennan, M.J., and Passik, S.D. (1996). Lymphoedema complicated by pain and psychological distress: A case with complex treatment needs. *J Pain Symptom Manage*, 12, 376–379.

5 Swarm, R., Karanikolas, M., and Cousins, M.J. (2004). Anaesthetic techniques for pain control. In Doyle, D., Hanks, G., Cherney, N., and Calman, K., eds. *Oxford textbook of palliative medicine*, 3rd edn, pp. 377–396. New York, Oxford University Press.

6 Hathaway, P.B., Mankoff, D.A., Maravilla, K.R., *et al.* (1999). Value of combining FDG PET and MR imaging in the evaluation of suspected recurrent local-regional breast cancer: Preliminary experience. *Radiology*, 210, 807–814.

7 Kori, S.H., Foley, K.M., and Posner, J.B. (1981). Brachial plexus lesions in patients with cancer: clinical findings in 100 cases. *Neurology*, 31, 45–50.

8 MacDonald, R.N., Hugi, M.R., Graydon, J.E., Beaulieu, M., *et al.* (1998). The management of chronic pain in patients with breast cancer. *Can Med Assoc J*, 158, 71–81.

9 World Health Organization (1986). *Cancer pain relief*. Geneva: WHO.

10 Bombardier, C. (2000). Comparison of upper gastrointestinal toxicity of rofecoxib and naproxen in patients with rheumatoid arthritis. *N Eng J Med*, 343, 1520–1528.

11 Fallon, M.T. (2000). Molecular genetics and palliative medicine: What is the link? *Pall Med*, 14, 1–2.

12 Fallon, M.T. (1997). Opioid rotation: Does it have a role? *Pall Med*, 11, 177–178.

13 Mercadante, S., Casuccio, A., Groff, L., *et al.* (2001). Switching from morphine to methadone to improve analgesia and tolerability in cancer patients. A prospective study. *J Clin Oncol*, 19, 2898–2904.

14 Ripamonti, C., Groff, L., Brunelli, C., *et al.* (1998). Switching from morphine to oral methadone in treating cancer pain: what is the equianalgesic dose ratio? *J Clin Oncol*, 16, 3216–3221.

15 Fitzgibbon, E.J., Hall, P., Schroder, C., Seely, J., and Viola, R. (2002). Low dose ketamine as an analgesic adjuvant in difficult pain syndromes: A strategy for conversion from parental to oral ketamine. *J Pain Symptom Manage*, 23, 165–170.

16 Robins, G. and Farr, P.M. (1997). Pain relief with Emla of ulcerating lesions in mycosis fungoides. *Br J Dermatol*, 136, 287.

17 Stein, C. (1995). The control of pain in peripheral tissue by opioids. *N Engl J Med*, 332, 1685–1690.

18 Flock, P. (2003). Pilot study to determine the effectiveness of diamorphine gel to control pressure ulcer pain. *J Pain Symptom Manage*, 25, 547–554.

19 Zeppeteela, G., Paul, J., and Ribeiro, M. (2003). Analgesic efficacy of morphine applied topically to painful ulcers. *J Pain Symptom Manage*, 25, 555–558.

20 Twillman, R.K., Long, T.D., Cathers, T.A., and Meuller, D.W. (1999). Treatment of painful skin ulcers with topical opioids. *J Pain Symptom Manage*, 17, 288–292.

21 Ellison, N., Loprinzi, C., Kugler, J., *et al.* (1997). Phase III placebo-controlled trial of capsaicin cream in the management of surgical neuropathic pain in cancer patients. *J Clin Oncol*, 15, 2974–2980.

22 Hill, D. (2003). Peripheral nerve blocks: practical aspects. In Breivik, H., Campbell, W., and Eccleston, C. eds. *Clinical pain management – practical applications and procedures*, pp. 197–222. London, Arnold.

23 Myers, D.P., Lema, M.J., De Leon-Casasola, O.A., and Bacon, D.R. (1993). Interpleural analgesia for the treatment of severe cancer pain in terminally ill patients. *J Pain Symptom Manage*, 8, 505–510.

24 Fishbain, D. (2000). Evidence-based data on pain relief with antidepressants. *Ann Medicine*, 32, 305–316.

25 Tremont-Lukats, I.W., Megeff, C., and Backonja, M.M. (2000). Anticonvulsants for neuropathic pin syndromes: Mechanisms of action and place in therapy. *Drugs*, 60, 1029–1052.

26 Grond, S., Radbruch, L., Meuser, T., Sabatowsku, R., Loick, G., and Lehmann, K.A. (1999). Assessment and treatment of neuropathic cancer pain following WHO guidelines. *Pain*, 79, 15–20.

27 Tarumi, Y., Watanabe, S., Bruera, E., and Ishitani, K. (2000). High-dose ketamine in the management of cancer-related neuropathic pain. *J Pain Symptom Manage*, 19, 405–407.

28 Kannan, T.R., Saxena, A., Bhatnagar, S., and Barry, A. (2002). Oral ketamine as an adjuvant to oral morphine for neuropathic pain in cancer patients. *J Pain Symptom Manage*, 23, 60–65.

29 Mercadante, S., Arcuri, E., Tirelli, W., and Casuccio, A. (2000). Analgesic effects of intravenous ketamine in cancer patients on morphine therapy: A randomized, controlled, double-blind, crossover, double-dose study. *J Pain Symptom Manage*, 20, 246–52.

30 Bruera, E., Ripamonti, C., Brenneis, C., Macmillan, K., and Hanson, J. (1992). A randomised double-blind crossover trial of intravenous lidocaine in the treatment of neuropathic cancer pain. *J Pain Symptom Manage*, 7, 138–140.

31 Chong, S., Bretscher, M., Maillard, J., *et al.* (1997). Pilot study evaluating local anaesthetics administered systemically for treatment of pain in patients with advanced cancer. *J Pain Symptom Manage*, 13, 112–117.

32 Brose, W.G. and Cousins, M.J. (1991). Subcutaneous lidocaine for the treatment of neuropathic cancer pain. *Pain*, 45, 145–148.

33 Dunlop, R.J., Hockley, J.M., Tate, T., and Turner, P. (1991). Flecainide in cancer nerve pain. *Lancet*, 337, 1347.

34 Lussier, D. and Portenoy, R.K. (2004). Adjuvant analgesics in pain management. In Doyle, D., Hanks, G., Cherney, N., and Calman, K., eds. *Oxford textbook of palliative medicine*, 3rd edn, pp. 349–378. New York, Oxford University Press.

35 Meier, T., Wasner, G., Faust, M., *et al.* (2003). Efficacy of lidocaine patch 5% in the treatment of focal peripheral neuropathic pain syndromes: a randomised, double-blind , placebo controlled study. *Pain*, 106, 151–158.

36 Devers, A. and Galer, B. (2000).Topical lidocaine patch relieves a variety of neuropathic pain conditions: An open-label study. *Clin J Pain*, 16, 205–208.

37 Rowbotham, M.C., Davies, P.C., and Fields, H.L. (1995). Topical lidocaine gel relieves postherpetic neuralgia. *Ann Neurology*, 37, 246–253.

38 Waldman, S. (2001). Brachial plexus block. In Waldman, S., ed. *Interventional pain management*, 2nd edn, pp. 382–387. Philadelphia, WB Saunders Company.

39 Vranken, J.H., van der Vegt, M.H., Zuurmond, W.W.A., Pijl, A.J., and Dzoljic, M. (2001). Continuous brachial plexus block at the cervical level using a posterior approach in the management of neuropathic cancer pain. *Regional Anaesthesia Pain Medicine*, 26, 572–575.

40 O'Leary, K.A., Yarussi, A.T., and Myers, D. (2001). Interpleural catheters: indications and techniques. In Waldman, S., ed. *Interventional pain management*, 2nd edn, pp. 409–414. Philadelphia, WB Saunders.

41 Hassenbusch, S.J. and Cherny, N.I. (2004). Neurosurgical approaches in palliative medicine. In Doyle, D., Hanks, G., Cherney, N., and Calman, K., eds. *Oxford textbook of palliative medicine*, 3rd edn, pp. 396–404. New York, Oxford University Press.

42 Portenoy, R., Forbes, K., Lussier, D., and Hanks, G. (2004). Difficult pain problems:an integrated approach. In Doyle, D., Hanks, G., Cherney, N., and Calman, K., eds. *Oxford textbook of palliative medicine*, 3rd edn, pp. 438–458. New York, Oxford University Press.

43 Twycross, R. (2000). Pain in lymphoedema. In Twycross, R., Jenns, K., and Todd, J. eds. *Lymphoedema*, pp. 68–88. Oxon, Radcliffe Medical Press.

44 Filshie, J. and Redman, D. (1985). Acupuncture and malignant pain problems. *Eur J Surg Oncol*, 11, 389–394.

45 Doyle, L., McClure, J., and Fisher, S. (2004). The contribution of physiotherapy to palliative medicine. In Doyle, D., Hanks, G., Cherney, N., and Calman, K., eds. *Oxford textbook of palliative medicine*, 3rd edn, pp. 1050–1056. New York, Oxford University Press.

46 Keeley, V. (2000). Oedema in advanced cancer. In Twycross, R., Jenns, K., and Todd, J. eds. *Lymphoedema*, pp. 338–358. Oxon, Radcliffe Medical Press.

47 Bray, J. and Cooper, J. (2004). The contribution to palliative medicine of allied health professions. In Doyle, D., Hanks, G., Cherney, N., and Calman, K., eds. *Oxford textbook of palliative medicine*, 3rd edn, pp. 1036–1040. New York, Oxford University Press.

48 Bercovitch, M. and Waller, A. (2004). Treating pain with transcutaneous electrical stimulation (TENS). In Doyle, D., Hanks, G., Cherney, N., and Calman, K., eds. *Oxford textbook of palliative medicine*, 3rd edn, pp. 405–9. New York, Oxford University Press.

49 Filshie, J., Scase, A., Ashley, S., and Hood, J. (1997). A study of the acupuncture effects on pain, anxiety and depression in patients with breast cancer (abstract). *Pain Society Meeting*.

50 Filshie, J. and Thompson, J. (2004). Acupuncture. In Doyle, D., Hanks, G., Cherney, N., and Calman, K., eds. *Oxford textbook of palliative medicine*, 3rd edn, pp. 410–424. New York, Oxford University Press.

51 **Maguire, P.** (1999). Late adverse psychological sequelae of breast cancer and its treatment. *Eur J Surg Oncol,* 25, 317–320.

52 **Cherny, N., Coyle, N., and Foley, K.** (1994). Suffering in the advanced cancer patient. Part 1: a definition and taxonomy. *J Pall Care,* 10, 57–70.

53 **Breitbart, W., Payne, D., and Passik, S.** (2004). Psychological and psychiatric interventions in pain control. In Doyle, D., Hanks, G., Cherney, N., and Calman, K., eds. *Oxford textbook of palliative medicine,* 3rd edn, pp. 424–438. New York, Oxford University Press.

54 **Vrkljan, B. and Miller-Polgar, J.** (2001). Meaning of occupational engagement in life-threatening illness: A qualitative pilot project. *Canadian J Occup Therapy,* 64, 237–246.

55 **Chalmers, K., Marles, S., Tataryn, D., Scott-Findlay, S., and Serfas, K.** (2003). Reports of information and support needs of daughters and sisters of women with breast cancer. *Eur J Cancer Care,* 12, 81–91.

# Chapter 3

# Psychological and social issues for patients with advanced breast cancer

Elizabeth A. Grunfeld

## Introduction

The diagnosis of a disease which has the potential to shorten an individual's life considerably will obviously raise a range of psychological and social issues. For some patients life may appear more valuable and worth fighting for, reflected perhaps in a desire for palliative chemotherapy. However, for other patients there may be a struggle to come to terms with a diagnosis of incurable disease and with the range of emotional responses that may accompany this situation. There is considerable research evidence from patients with early breast cancer that the diagnosis of the disease and the accompanying treatment are associated with psychological distress and social morbidity. There have been fewer studies that have examined psychosocial issues relevant to metastatic breast cancer and to palliative chemotherapy; however, interest and research in this area has increased over recent years. Such research can tell us much about the needs of advanced breast cancer patients and help clinicians to understand how to support patients in this stage of the disease. Psychosocial issues are becoming increasingly important in oncology and are central to palliative care, and this chapter will focus on some of the main psychosocial issues among patients with advanced breast cancer and will present evidence and guidelines where they exist.

## Psychological distress and psychiatric morbidity

Psychological distress, including depression and anxiety, does not necessarily emerge in patients with advanced breast cancer.[1] There are, however, peak times or 'crisis points' when psychological distress may occur and such crisis points include the development of metastases and entering the terminal phase of illness.[2] There are also a number of disease and treatment-related factors that might lead to these emotional responses, including the side-effects of treatment and the disability and symptoms that might accompany advancing disease.[3] In fact, the association between poor performance status and clinical depression is a consistent finding in the research literature.[4-6] A further consistent finding is the role of age, with greater physical and mental distress being apparent among patients below 50 years of age.[7,8]

Not surprisingly, the experience of anxiety and depression are known to have a significant negative impact on quality of life. Of concern, however, is that an estimated 80% of the psychological and psychiatric morbidity that develops in cancer patients may go unrecognized[9] and a similar pattern is thought to exist among patients with advanced breast cancer. One of the main reasons that distress among these patients may go unrecognized is that patients may choose not to disclose their feelings due to concerns about wasting the clinician's time or because they feel that they are in some way to blame for how they are feeling.[10] Approximately 25% of patients with advanced breast cancer may have clinically significant anxiety or depression,[6] which is much higher than the incidence observed in the healthy population. Evidence is conflicting regarding whether patients with terminal illness are more likely to experience anxiety or depression or both.[6, 11] The Royal College of Radiologists recommend that metastatic breast cancer patients have a formal assessment not only of physical symptoms but also of psychosocial needs.[12] However, the difficulties associated with carrying out such assessments are recognized and the College recommend that all staff involved in the management of such patients receive appropriate training to enable the early identification of psychological and psychiatric problems.

The need for patients to have their psychological needs assessed and managed at every stage of the 'cancer journey' from diagnosis to palliation has also been set out in the NICE guidance; it will require all multidisciplinary teams, in cancer or palliative care, to have staff with a range of psychological expertise to ensure that this is accomplished.[13] All teams will need to have a clinician who has specialist psychological training. A four-level model of professional psychological assessment has been proposed and the recommendation is that such a framework should be implemented in each Cancer Network. The model aims to encompass the diversity of psychological expertise and skills that might be provided by the different professional disciplines that form a palliative care team (Table 3.1).

**Table 3.1** NICE model of psychological assessment and support

| | |
|---|---|
| Level 1 | Effective information giving, communication and general psychological care (given by all of the multidisciplinary team) |
| Level 2 | Crisis management and simple psychological interventions (given by all of the multidisciplinary team) |
| Level 3 | Counselling and psychotherapy, formal and specialist psychological support (given by counsellors and psychological therapists) |
| Level 4 | Psychiatric and specialized medical psychotherapeutic interventions (given by a range of psychological therapists, e.g. clinical psychologists, psychiatrists, medical psychotherapists, counsellors, and others) |

## Screening for depression

In the physically healthy population, depression is diagnosed if patients have a persistent low mood and at least four other identifying symptoms present most of the day for the preceding 2 weeks. These symptoms include psychomotor retardation, changes in sleep and appetite, and fatigue. However, these symptoms could be present in patients with advanced breast cancer not because they are depressed but rather due to metastatic disease or its treatment and therefore such symptoms may not be helpful in identifying the presence of depression. It is preferable, therefore, to employ measures of anxiety and depression that exclude the somatic symptoms that patients with advanced breast cancer might experience as part of their disease or as side-effects of their treatment.

The Present State Examination (PSE) is a valid tool that generates information from which it is possible to make a psychiatric diagnosis using the standard classification of the International Classification of Diseases.[14] The PSE comprises two parts; part one examines neurotic symptoms, eating disorders, drug and alcohol misuse, and also includes a screening tool to determine whether to use part two, which focuses on psychotic experiences, speech, and behaviour. Although the PSE is a deemed to be a robust and valid tool its major drawback, for use in the clinic, is that interviewers must be appropriately trained and supervised.[15]

There are a number of well-validated short questionnaire measures, such as the Hospital Anxiety and Depression Scale and the General Health Questionnaire.[16,17] Both are quick to administer and easy to score and interpret. However, from a clinical perspective, these measures cannot replace a full mental state examination and it is recommended that all staff who are regularly involved in the psychological care of patients with advanced breast cancer obtain full training in undertaking such an interview. It has been recommended that physicians without structured training be encouraged to assess and probe their patients regarding cognitive symptoms such as anhedonia, guilt, suicidal thinking, and hopelessness.[18] Whether or not to initiate pharmacological treatment for depression often depends on assessing the probability that the patient will recover spontaneously in the next 2 to 4 weeks as well as the severity and duration of the symptoms. Antidepressants are commonly prescribed in the palliative care setting for cases of depression and many palliative care teams and specialist palliative care units (hospices) have suitably qualified and experienced staff to undertake this work. However, studies have shown that the treatment of major depression is optimized by a combination of pharmacotherapy, psychotherapy, and increased social support, so even when pharmacological treatments are in place a referral to psychotherapy or supportive counselling should be considered. Therefore it is important to be aware of the liaison psychiatry, counselling, and family support services available in your establishment or locality for patients with advanced breast cancer.

## Checklist

- ◆ Depression is not necessarily an outcome of metastatic breast cancer.
- ◆ Many cases of depression may go unrecognized and therefore screening is advised.
- ◆ Measures should exclude somatic symptoms that might be indicative of metastatic disease.
- ◆ Staff who are regularly involved with the care of patients with advanced breast cancer should receive appropriate training in the identification of psychological distress.
- ◆ Treatment of major depression is optimized by a combination of pharmacotherapy and psychotherapy and appropriate social support.

## Decision making for treatment

Palliative chemotherapy may be prescribed for a range of reasons including prolongation of life, management of existing symptoms, delaying the onset of new symptoms, improving patient mobility, and possibly to maintain a sense of hope.[19,20] However, decisions regarding the management of advanced breast cancer are often complex; this complexity is due, in part, to the absence of a cure. There is also a concern that patients' understanding of the outcomes of chemotherapy may be overly optimistic.[21] Patients with advanced cancer may be willing to accept anticancer treatment even when there is only a small chance, and a potentially short duration, of benefit.[20] Patients may be more likely to accept palliative chemotherapy in situations where health care professionals and healthy individuals expect them to decline.[22] Some patients with advanced breast cancer may also pursue anticancer treatments without a clear understanding of their prognosis and management options.[21,23]

## Provision of information

It is important to ensure that patients receive appropriate information about the prognosis of their cancer and the likely outcomes of treatment. By involving patients in the clinical decision-making process regarding the management of their disease it is possible to facilitate the process of informed decision making. It is possible to improve this process by providing patients with a checklist of the sort of questions that they can ask a clinician during their consultation. As well as ensuring that patients are aware of the sort of questions to ask it is also important to ensure that they remember the answers to those questions and any additional information that they are provided with. At a difficult time, such as a consultation about palliative treatment, patients may not assimilate and remember what is said to them. Patient recall can, however, be improved by the provision of an audiotape of the consultation. Perhaps more useful would be a written summary of the topics and options discussed as well as the outcome and reasons for that outcome. Such an *aide-mémoire* may ease some of the anxiety accompanying decision making at such a stressful time and may also serve to improve patient satisfaction with the chosen treatment.[24] Finally, it is necessary to check that patients have understood the information provided; patient understanding is checked in only 10% of consultations.[25]

## The patient's role in the decision-making process

The Royal College of Radiologists[12] recommend that women with breast cancer be offered the opportunity to participate in decision making regarding their treatment options and this is also a requirement of the recent NICE guidance.[13] However, providing detailed information to those who do not want it and imposing choice on those who would prefer that their doctor assume responsibility for making treatment decisions is likely to be harmful.[26, 27] A significant proportion of patients prefer to relinquish decisional control, particularly if faced with a poor prognosis.[28] Therefore it is important to remember two fundamental issues that are important when discussing complex treatment options with patients. Firstly, the information provided to the patient should match their information needs, both in terms of the amount provided and the type of information desired. Secondly, the patients should be encouraged to participate in the decision-making process to whatever degree is acceptable to them (which may mean that some patients may choose to opt out of the decision making process).

The association between the role patients wish to play in decision-making and their desire for information, however, is not straightforward.[27] Active patients (those who desire an active role in decision making) are known to desire more detailed information about their diagnosis and treatment options than passive patients. However, there are individual and psychosocial factors that also influence preference for involvement in the decision-making process. Although assumptions should not be made, there is evidence that younger patients prefer to take an active role in decisions about their care; 87% of patients under 40 express a desire to participate, compared to 51% of patients over the age of 60.[29] Furthermore, it is important to remember that clinicians are not able to consistently predict the decision-making preferences of their patients[30] and often underestimate patients' desire for information.[31] Establishing the patient's decision-making preferences and information needs could help improve the communication process between clinician and patient. This could be facilitated by simply asking the patient how much information they require or by checking at the end of the consultation that enough detail and information has been provided. Trying to determine how involved a patient wishes to be in the decision-making process can be more difficult. It is possible to simply ask the patient but often patients may not express their true views for fear of offending a clinician who they know is trying to prolong their life or reduce their suffering. It is possible to use a decisional preferences scale, which aims to elicit how involved the patient would like to be with options ranging from leaving all the decisions to the clinician to fully making the decision themselves.[32]

Finally, the relationship between a clinician and the patient should not be underestimated. Results from research with early breast cancer patients suggest that the relationship between the physician and patient is as important to patients in their decision to accept chemotherapy, as are their concerns about side-effects and recurrence.[33] Providing patients had a good relationship with their clinician then they were content to accept the oncologist's recommendation and were confident that they would receive the most appropriate treatment.

## Checklist

- Patients vary in their preference for information about their disease and treatment with regards to participation in the decision making process.
- It is important to ascertain the patient's desire to participate in the decision process.
- It is important to check that the patient has received all the information they desire and has understood the information provided.

## The effects of treatment

There is great variability in the way in which women with advanced breast cancer cope with their treatment. Treatment for breast cancer can limit a woman's ability to perform daily functions and may also have implications for perceptions of body image and sexuality. Research into early breast cancer has shown that it is not safe to assume that lumpectomy will result in less distress than more radical surgery (mastectomy)[34] as the effects of other treatments (such as radiotherapy) may be perceived by some patients as highly stressful. This could be due to the demands that regular visits place on everyday function but may also be due to symptoms, such as fatigue or nausea, which can be induced by treatment. There is also evidence to suggest that palliative chemotherapy administered in hospital may be perceived as more distressing than chemotherapy administered in the patient's home.[11] It is important that the patient's concerns are discussed in relation to the choice of treatment and that information is provided that prepares the patient for the impact of treatment.

Although palliative chemotherapy may prolong the life of a patient with advanced breast cancer by several months or even years,[35] the outcomes of chemotherapy cannot be guaranteed. There is evidence to suggest that even objective disease response does not necessarily lead to improved quality of life as reported by the patient.[36] Furthermore, the chemotherapy itself may be associated with side-effects such as nausea, hair loss, and fatigue which can negatively impact on the patient's quality of life.[37, 38] These side-effects may also influence the way in which a patient perceives the chemotherapy. For example in a consecutive series of 155 women with advanced breast cancer undergoing first-line chemotherapy, 26% of patients reported feeling better, 19% reported feeling the same, and 22% felt worse than they did before treatment.[39] The same study found that half the patients who survived to the final interview reported that the treatment had been very or moderately worthwhile. However, the same number of patients reported that the treatment had been only a little or not at all worthwhile. It is important that patients are aware of the impact of side-effects that can accompany palliative chemotherapy and that they are aware of alternatives to anticancer treatments, such as supportive care alone or specialist palliative care alone.

## Checklist

+ Patients' goals need to be at the centre of any management plan.
+ Clear, unambiguous advice about the effect of any chemotherapy offered on symptom control, and quality and length of life is needed to enable patients to make informed choices about the sort of care they want.
+ Patients should be provided with information about the side-effects of *all* treatments that they are offered.
+ Patients' desires and concerns about their treatment and care need to be ascertained.
+ Patients should be made aware of the alternatives to anticancer treatment.

## Social issues

The incidence of social isolation, where an individual chooses not to mix in the mainstream of society, among patients with advanced breast cancer is lower than that observed among patients with primary or recurrent breast cancer. There may, however, be a reduction in the social interaction of patients with advanced breast cancer due to the physical and social changes that occur with advancing disease – fatigue, for example, may limit social life, patients often retire from work and can no longer maintain the other roles that they have managed before. Some patients may also lack adequate social support structures, both in terms of the size of their support network and the quality of that support. This may be particularly true in the case of the elderly. Although the degree of social support a cancer patient has is not related to survival, it is known to have a role in the psychological adjustment of patients to their diagnosis and also to be associated with the occurrence of depression. Research has suggested that for patients with advanced breast cancer perceived social support is influenced by a belief that others are there for the patient and that they do not create additional stress for the patient.[40]

However, one of the most significant issues for patients with advanced cancer is the concern about the future of their family. One way that patients cope with this is by actively making sure that family members are equipped to cope after their death.[41] Family members, while trying to provide support to the patient, may themselves be under considerable strain as they attempt to cope with the patient's advancing disease. A possible outcome is that both the patient and family members avoid discussing their emotions and psychological needs, which can lead to a sense of isolation for all the individuals involved. If patients do withdraw in this way there is the potential for depression to develop.

It is essential to ensure that the children of patients with advanced breast cancer – not only the very young but also teenagers and younger adults or others who are vulnerable, perhaps because of learning difficulties or previous bereavement – are kept in touch (in appropriate detail) and feel able to ask about what is happening to their parent. Specialist palliative care teams and services are used to advising on this sort of issue and offering help where it is needed. Complex grief in this group can lead to depression and difficulty with intimate relationships in adult life.

There is growing concern about the needs of the family and caregivers of patients with advanced cancer. In addition to the occupational and economic burdens that may result from adopting a caring role, recent research has shown that caregivers' depression and perceived burden increases as the patient's functional status declines.[42] The importance of involving significant others in the patient's treatment and care is well recognized as is identifying a primary caregiver for issues relating to terminal disease. However, recently there has also been a call for clinicians to become more aware of the concept of the 'family' in a climate of growth of non-traditional households. This places a responsibility on the clinician to ensure that anyone that the patient chooses is included in the care and treatment process.

## Checklist

- ◆ It is important to identify the patient's degree of support, particularly among the elderly.
- ◆ The needs and concerns of family and carers should be addressed.
- ◆ It is important to identify and be inclusive of non-traditional 'family' structures.

# Interventions

## Pharmacological interventions

The National Cancer Institute states that pharmacological therapy is indicated in a number of cases of depression in patients with cancer and is efficacious in the treatment of depressive symptoms. There has also been shown to be a measurable improvement in quality of life following treatment with antidepressants. It is estimated that 25% of all cancer patients experience depressive symptoms; however, only around 2% will receive antidepressant medication.[43] The types of medications generally used to treat depression in patients with cancer are either the selective serotonin reuptake inhibitors (SSRIs), such as fluoxetine, or the tricyclic antidepressants (TCAs), such as mianserin. Generally, a long latency period is observed (3 to 6 weeks) between starting the antidepressant medication and a therapeutic response. In many cases treatment begins at low dose (which may help avoid initial side-effects), followed by gradual dose titration until the optimum response is achieved for that individual. However, a recent systematic review concluded that there were too few adequate studies in this field to draw clear conclusions about the best management of depression in a palliative care setting.[44]

## Psychological

The systematic review of treatment of depression in palliative care also found that there were no randomized control trials that specifically assessed psychotherapy for patients with depression.[44] However, despite the paucity of adequate studies, the National Cancer Institute acknowledges that depressive symptoms are often well managed by a combination of crisis intervention, brief supportive psychotherapy, and cognitive behavioural techniques. Patients are usually required to attend for several sessions (often between three and ten) the aims of which are to improve coping skills and to reshape negative or self-defeating thoughts. Such sessions may also help by providing information and clarifying concerns about the illness and its treatment and to assure patients about the role of the palliative care team.

## Social

Support groups can provide useful social support networks for patients. In addition, interventions based on a support group format have been shown to have positive effects on mood disturbance, quality of life, and positive immune responses. Although it might not always be possible for palliative care patients to access support groups it is important to be aware of appropriate groups and to consider the use of informal groups within a hospice setting.

## Checklist

◆ Few studies have adequately examined the best management of depression.
◆ Antidepressants have been shown to be efficacious in the treatment of depressive symptoms.

◆ Psychological interventions can help patients improve coping skills and can help tackle negative thoughts.

◆ Formal and informal support groups may have positive effects on a patient's mood and quality of life.

## Conclusion

The psychological and social issues that accompany the diagnosis and treatment of advanced breast cancer are both complex and varied. Interest in this area has increased over the years, both with regards to research and in the clinical setting. There are now evidence-based guidelines available to help manage the psycho-social distress that may accompany advanced breast cancer. Clinicians need training and the support of psychological and palliative care services in order to identify and effectively manage these issues when they arise.

## References

1 Brugha, T. (1993). Depression in the terminally ill. *Br J Hopsital Med*, 10, 175–181.

2 Lloyd-Williams, M. and Friedman, T. (2001). Depression in palliative care patients – a prospective study. *Eur J Cancer Care*, 10, 270–274.

3 Greer, S. and Silberfarb, P.M. (1982). Psychological concomitants of cancer: current state of research. *Psychol Med*, 12, 563–573.

4 Bukberg, J., Penman, D., and Holland, J. (1984). Depression in hospitalised cancer patients. *Psychosom Med*, 46, 199–212.

5 Hopwood, P., Howell, A., and McGuire, P. (1991). Screening for psychiatric morbidity in patients with advanced breast cancer: validation of two self-report questionnaires. *Br J Cancer*, 64, 353–356.

6 Pinder, K.L., Ramirez, A.J., Black, M.E., Richards, M.A., Gregory, W.M., and Rubens, R.D. (1993). Psychiatric disorder in patients with advanced breast cancer: prevalence and associated factors. *Eur J Cancer*, 29A, 524–527.

7 Harrison, J. and Maguire, P. (1994). Predictors of psychiatric morbidity in cancer patients. *Br J Psychiatry*, 165, 593–598.

8 Parle, M., Gallagher, J., Gray, C., Akers, G., and Liebert, B. (2001). From evidence to practice: factors affecting the specialist breast nurse's detection of psychological morbidity in women with breast cancer. *Psycho-Oncol*, 10, 503–510.

9 Magiure, P. (1985). Psychological morbidity associated with cancer and cancer treatment. *Clinics Oncol*, 4, 559–575.

10 Maguire, P. and Howell, A. Improving the psychological care of cancer patients. In Houses, A., Mayou, R., and Mallinson, C., eds. (1995) *Psychiatric aspects of physical disease*, pp. 41–54. London, Royal College of Physicians and Royal College of Psychiatrists.

11 Payne, S.A. (1992). A study of quality of life in cancer patients receiving palliative chemotherapy. *Soc Sci Med*, 35, 1505–1509.

12 Royal College of Radiologists (2002). *Guidelines on the non-surgical management of breast cancer*. London, Royal College of Radiologists.

13 NICE (2004). *Improving supportive and palliative care for adults with cancer*. London, National Institute for Clinical Excellence.

14 Wing, J.A. (1976). Technique for studying psychiatric morbidity in inpatient and outpatient series and in general population samples. *Psychol Med*, 6, 665–671.

15 Lesage, A.D., Cope, S.J., and Pezeshgi, S. (1991). Assessing the needs for care of non-psychotic patients. A trial with a new standardized procedure. *Soc Psychiatry Psychiatr Epidemiol*, 26, 281–286.

16 Zigmond, A.S. and Snaith, R.P. (1983). The hospital anxiety and depression scale. *Acta Psychiatr Scand*, 67, 361–370.

17 Goldberg, D. (1992). *General Health Questionnaire (GHQ-12)*. Windsor, NFER-NELSON.

18 Passik, S.D., Dugan, W., McDonald, M.V., Rosenfeld, B., Theobald, D.E., and Edgerton, S. (1998). Oncologists' recognition of depression in their patients with cancer. *J Clin Oncol*, 16, 1594–1600.

19 Rubens, R.D., Towlson, K.E., Ramirez, A.J., Coltrat, S., Slevin, M.L., Terrell, C., and Timothy, A.R. (1992). Appropriate chemotherapy for palliating advanced cancer. *BMJ*, 304, 35–40.

20 Grunfeld, E.A., Ramirez, A.J., Maher, E.J., Peach, D., Young, T., Albery, I.P., and Richards, M.A. (2001). Chemotherapy for advanced breast cancer: what influences oncologists' decision making? *Br J Cancer*, 84, 1172–1178.

21 Weeks, J.C., Cook, E.F., O'Day, S.J., Peterson, L.M., Wenger, N., Reding, D., Harrell, F.E., Kussin, P., Dawson, N.V., Connors, A.F., Lynn, J., and Phillips, R.S. (1998). Relationship between cancer patients' predictions of prognosis and their treatment preferences. *JAMA*, 279, 1709–1714.

22 Balmer, C.E., Thomas, P., and Osborne, R.J. (2001). Who wants second-line palliative chemotherapy? *Psycho-Oncol*, 10, 410–418.

23 Gattellari, M., Voigt, K.J., Butow, P.N., and Tattersall, M.H.N. (2002). When the treatment goal is not the cure: are cancer patients equipped to make informed decisions? *J Clin Oncol*, 20, 503–513.

24 Bruera, E., Pituskin, E., Calder, K., Neumann, C.M., and Hanson, J. (1999). The addition of an audiocassette recording of a consultation to written recommendations for patients with advanced cancer. A randomised controlled trial. *Cancer*, 86, 2420–2425.

25 Tattersall, M.H., Gattellari, M., Voigt, K., and Butow, P.N. (2002). When the treatment goal is not cure: are patients informed adequately? *Support Care Cancer*, 10, 314–321.

26 Tobias, J.S. and Souhami, R.L. (1993). Fully informed consent can be needlessly cruel. *BMJ*, 307, 1199–1201.

27 Fallowfield, L. (2001). Participation of patients in decisions about treatment for cancer. *BMJ*, 323, 1144.

28 Guadagnoli, E. and Ward, P. (1998). Patient participation in decision-making. *Soc Sci Medicine*, 47, 329–339.

29 Cassileth, B.R., Zupkis, R.V., Sutton-Smith, K., and March, V. (1980). Information and participation preferences among cancer patients. *Ann Intern Med*, 92, 832–836.

30 Bruera, E., Sweeney, C., Calder, K., Palmer, L., and Benisch-Tolley, S. (2001). Patient preferences versus physician perceptions of treatment decisions in cancer care. *J Clin Oncol*, 19, 2883–2885.

31 Jenkins, V., Fallowfield, L., and Saul, J. (2001). Information needs of patients with cancer: results of a large study of UK cancer centres. *Br J Cancer*, 84, 48–51.

32 Degner, L.F. and Sloan, J.A. (1992). Decision making during serious illness: what role do patients really want to play? *J Clin Epidemiol*, 45, 941–950.

33 Henman, M.J., Butow, P.N., Brown, R.F., Boyle, F., and Tattersall, M.H.N. (2002). Lay constructions of decision-making in cancer. *Psycho-Oncol*, 11, 295–306.

34 Fallowfield, L.J., Baum, M., and Maguire, G.P. (1986). Effects of breast conservation on psychological morbidity associated with diagnosis and treatment of early breast cancer. *BMJ*, 293,1331–1334.

35 Cardoso, F., Di Leo, A., Lohrisch, C., Bernard, C., Ferreira, F., and Piccart, M.J. (2002). Second and subsequent lines of chemotherapy for metastatic breast cancer: what did we learn from the last two decades? *Ann Oncol*, 13, 197–207.

36 Michael, M. and Tannock, I.F. (1998). Measuring health-related quality of life in clinical trials that evaluate the role of chemotherapy in cancer treatment. *Can Med Assoc J*, 158, 1727–1734.

37 Dodwell, D.J. (1998). Adjuvant cytotoxic chemotherapy for early breast cancer: doubts and decisions. *Lancet*, 351, 1506–1507.

38 Porzsolt, F. and Tannock, I. (1993). Goals of palliative chemotherapy. *J Clin Oncol*, 11, 378–381.

39 Ramirez, A.J., Towlson, K.E., Leaning, M.S., Richards, M.A., and Rubens, R.D. (1998). Do patients with advanced breast cancer benefit from chemotherapy? *Br J Cancer*, 78, 1488–1494.

40 Koopman, C., Hermanson, K., Diamond, S., Angell, K., and Spiegal, D. (1998). Social support, life stress, pain and emotional adjustment to advanced breast cancer. *Psycho-Oncol*, 7, 101–111.

41 Wainstock, J.M. (1991). Breast cancer: psychosocial consequences for the patient. *Seminars Oncol Nursing*, 7, 207–215.

42 Grunfeld, E., Coyle, D., Whelan, T., Clinch, J., Reyno, L., Earle, C.C., Willan, A., Viola, R., Coristine, M., Janz, T., and Glossop, R. (2004). Family caregiver burden: results of a longitudinal study of breast cancer patients and their principal caregivers. *Can Med Assoc J*, 170, 1795–1801.

43 Stiefel, F., Die Trill, M., Berney, A., Olarte, J., and Razavi, D. (2001). Depression in palliative care: apragmatic report from the Expert Group of the Association for Palliative Care. *Support Care Cancer*, 9, 477–488.

44 Lan Ly, K., Chidgey, J., Addington-Hall, J., and Hotopf, M. (2002). Depression in palliative care: a systematic review. Part 2. Treatment. *Palliative Medicine*, 16, 279–284.

## Chapter 4

# The management of odours and wounds in advanced local disease

Kathryn G. Froiland

## Introduction

Malignant cutaneous wounds are skin lesions resulting from tumour infiltration of the epithelium, and the lymph and blood vessels supporting the epithelium. They may occur as primary skin lesions or as a result of metastasis from the primary tumour. Appearance of these lesions varies in colour, contour, presence of sinus tracts or fistulae, and depth of tissue involvement. Commonly associated symptoms are pain, drainage, bleeding, odour, infection, necrosis, pruritis, and friability of surrounding tissue. Chronic malignant wounds can be emotionally distressing as they represent a visible and constant reminder of the presence of cancer and its failure to respond to treatment. Living with a cutaneous malignant wound may incur personal, social, and financial losses, with associated changes in self-concept, roles, activities, and care requirements. The care of a patient with this type of wound requires a sensitive approach by the interdisciplinary palliative care team. The patient's care providers must also be included and supported during this time of both physical and emotional stress.

Scientific research supports evidence-based practice in managing chronic wounds of multiple origins. Cutaneous malignant wound management is guided by these standards of treatment. In recent years, a growing body of anecdotal clinical experience in this type of wound management has been published. Awareness of the challenges in cutaneous malignant wound management by health-care professionals has long been appreciated. It appears that there is a developing consensus in assessment and management of these especially unique and demanding wounds and the environment in which they exist.

The occurrence of cutaneous metastasis from solid tumours ranges from 5 to 10% of all cancer patients. Women with breast cancer are the most frequently affected, in the range of 18.5 to 50%.[1] Cutaneous malignant wounds present more often in recurrent disease. Healing potential is dependent on the responsiveness of the primary tumour to treatment. As the tumour becomes less responsive to treatment, often the healing potential of the wound deteriorates. The wound becomes chronic in nature, requiring management of symptoms without realistic hope for closure of the wound.

## Assessment

Wounds do not exist in isolation. The health-care professional must determine the wound's cause, the patient's underlying medical condition and treatment status, and the history of the wound and its management to date. This information aids in classification, identifies previous unsuccessful management attempts, and may explain delayed healing and or progression. *Remember to position the patient comfortably and medicate if necessary prior to wound assessment and care.* Wound assessment and documentation should include the following aspects:

♦ degree of tissue layer destruction and colour;
♦ anatomic location;
♦ length, width, depth, and tunnelling using consistent units of measure;
♦ appearance of the wound bed and surrounding skin;
♦ drainage and bleeding – specifying amount, colour, consistency, odour;
♦ pain or tenderness of wound and surrounding skin;
♦ temperature of tissue.[2]

Potential for further breakdown of the surrounding skin should be assessed so as to plan preventive measures. Excessive dryness, moisture, or non-viable tissue may result in pruritis, pain, and loss of skin integrity. Assessment of the wound for the presence of foreign objects is advised, as these materials may cause infection or delay healing.

Haisfield–Wolfe and Baxendale–Cox have developed a staging system for malignant cutaneous wounds. Although not universally implemented, it may provide a useful tool for assessment and consistent documentation:

**Stage I:** Closed, dry wound that is red/pink in colour.

**Stage I-N:** Wound that occasionally opens superficially to drain, then closes again. The wound colour is red/pink and drainage may be clear or purulent. These wounds may be *painful*.

**Stage II:** Partial-thickness skin loss involving dermal and epidermal tissue. The wound colour is red/pink and drainage may be serosanguinous or sanguinous. These wounds are likely to be *painful* and tend to be *malodorous*.

**Stage III:** Full thickness skin loss involving subcutaneous tissue. The wound colour may be red/pink or yellow, and drainage is purulent or serosanguinous. These wounds are likely to be *painful* and tend to be *malodorous*.

**Stage IV:** Full thickness skin loss with invasion into deep anatomic tissues and structures. Tunnelling is often present. The wound colour may be red/pink or yellow, and drainage is serosanguinous, sanguinous, or purulent. *Pain is likely,* and the wound tends to be *malodorous*.[3]

Consultation with a plastic / reconstructive surgeon may be of benefit to assess and potentially treat wounds involving underlying tissues. If tissue involvement is deemed to be too deep and therefore not amenable to surgical intervention, this finding will guide the care planner in planning subsequent wound management. Cutaneous malignant wounds present unique challenges due to their complexity and ever-changing characteristics. The wound must be managed within the context of the patient's overall plan of care. For these reasons, it is recommended that assessment and management is carried out by a wound care expert who is also experienced in the care of oncology patients. Further information may be obtained from the website of the Wound Ostomy and Incontinence Nurses Society (www.wocn.org).

# Management

Wound closure and healing are the ultimate goals of all types of wound management protocols. However, these goals may be unattainable when caring for a patient with a cutaneous malignant wound. Immunosuppression, nutritional compromise, infection, and unresponsive disease will delay or prevent healing. Aiming at the prevention of further progression and maintaining the existing wound and surrounding tissue may be more realistic.

Sometimes it is necessary to admit patients with very extensive or neglected (often concealed) wounds to give the most effective care to the patient (and her carers) and to bring about the best improvement possible. Occasionally, patients will need periodic readmission to continue wound care. In addition to the extent, moistness, and malodour of wounds accompanying concealed disease, the relatives are often very shocked and distressed when they find out what has been hidden from them and the implications for the diagnosis of advanced, incurable disease.

Serial photography is a commonly used mechanism to document progression to healing of wounds. In the palliative care setting it may be inappropriate, as documentation of worsening disease may be distressing to the patient and family. Photography is of questionable value in the patient with aggressive end-stage cancer. The use of photography should be evaluated openly, and guided by the patient's wishes.

## Individual treatment plans

Treatment plans must be individualized and include goals agreed upon by the patient, family, and care provider. The plan of care should consider emotional and social issues of the patient and care provider. Dressing changes should be as pain-free as possible for the patient. The patient should be positioned and supported comfortably following adequate premedication with a pain-relieving agent. The dressing removal and reapplication procedure should involve a minimum of steps to be achievable by the care provider. All concerns should be addressed in planning wound care so it does not overburden the patient and family, especially if a family member will be performing wound care.

## Other techniques

Treatment options are aimed at the underlying pathology and may include radiation therapy, chemotherapy, hormonal therapy, surgery, cryotherapy, or laser therapy.[4] Wounds may cause embarrassment and become socially isolating. The care provider must convey an attitude that allays feelings of rejection, shame, or disgust. Topical wound care is focused on control of symptoms of pain, bleeding, odour, and exudate.

## Managing odour

Odour is one of the most distressing symptoms for the patient to cope with. This concern should be addressed even when others cannot detect it. Necrotic tissue, infected tissue, or saturated dressings are sources of odour. There exist several methods of debridement to remove necrotic, devitalized tissue. Surgical or sharp debridement is the fastest method. It is invasive, may require anaesthesia, and should not be done if vasculature of the cutaneous tumour places the patient at risk for excessive bleeding. Licensing regulations and institutional policies require that a trained wound care professional perform this type of debridement. Mechanical debridement involves physical force to remove debris and necrotic tissue. It cannot discriminate between viable and non-viable tissue. Although commonly used in the past, wet-to-dry dressings are not recommended as they cause pain, bleeding, and tissue damage upon removal. Enzymatic debridement utilizes enzymes to dissolve necrotic tissue from the wound. Topical gels and solutions are directly applied to the eschar or applied following scoring of the eschar to allow penetration into the tissue. Enzymes are categorized as collagenases, fibrinolytics, and proteolytics. Autolytic debridement is a process that creates a moist environment allowing the wound bed to rid itself of dead tissue by endogenous proteolytic enzymes and phagocytic cells present in the wound and its drainage. Creation of this environment is achieved by application of an occlusive, semiocclusive, or moisture interactive dressing and/or an autolytic debriding gel directly applied to the wound surface. This process is potentially more time consuming; however, it can be effective and less traumatic than surgical, sharp, or mechanical methods. Biological (larvae therapy) debridement has resurfaced as a method useful in digesting necrotic tissue and pathogens. Consideration of this method may be appropriate when surgical debridement is not an option.

## Cleaning the wound

Warmed saline is the preferred cleansing solution for chronic wound care. It cleans the wound gently without harming viable tissue. It can be applied via soaked gauze or by irrigating by pouring solution, using a spray bottle or piston syringe. Pressure of 5–8 psi is adequate for cleansing, although 5–15 psi may be necessary to remove thick exudate. Devices delivering higher pressures should be avoided as they may cause tissue damage and bleeding. Use of commercial wound cleansing products and antiseptic agents are controversial. They require significant dilution to maintain phagocytic function and white blood cell viability. Guidelines can be found online through the National Guidelines Clearinghouse (www.guidelines.gov). Saline remains accepted as readily available, comforting, inexpensive, and harmless to the wound bed.

## Wound infection

Wounds are usually contaminated by surface aerobic pathogens. Malignant wounds may become infected (greater than $10^5$ colony-forming units of bacteria) by bacteria that may or may not be normal flora. Odour is often associated with anaerobic infection and should be treated with systemic antibiotics if the wound shows signs of infection such as cellulitis, septicaemia, or osteomyelitis. If infection appears to be superficial, topical antibiotics will decrease bacterial burden, wound odour, and exudate. Metronidazole has been used systemically and topically to control odour cause by anaerobic infection, including *Bacteroides* species. Oral doses of 200–400 mg bid for 10 days or topical application of 0.75–1.0% gel may be helpful in controlling odour. Crushing oral tablets into a powder form or dissolving the powder into solution can be a less costly alternative to the gel for topical application.[1] Chlorophyll-containing ointments or oral tablets may also offer odour control. Other topical low-cost options include the application of plain live yogurt or buttermilk for 15 min and then rinse off, four times per day. Sugar paste and honey have been cited as additional alternatives for odour control.[1]

## Dressings

Odour may also be caused by saturated dressings that are not changed frequently. Commercially available activated charcoal dressings are designed for malodorous wounds. Direct application is appropriate for scantily draining wounds. Highly exudative wounds require absorptive dressings applied to the wound surface, with the charcoal dressing applied as the secondary dressing. All edges should be secured to intact surrounding skin or protective barrier. Silver dressings can provide odour control, decrease bacterial burden, and can be removed atraumatically. A less expensive alternative method to be considered is the use of charcoal sheets from a pet store. Wound gel or hydrogel is applied to the wound surface, and covered by a non-adherent dressing or gauze. The charcoal sheet should then be placed. Cover the layers with an absorptive dressing and secure with non-traumatizing tape, roll gauze, or elastic netting material.[5]

The wound shape and volume of exudate must be matched to the dressing chosen for containment. Changing dressings more than twice daily can be burdensome for the care provider. Alginate, hydrofiber, or foam dressings absorb higher volumes of drainage than hydrocolloids or gauze. Collection of very heavily exudative wound drainage may be accomplished by using a drainable ostomy or wound drainage collecting device. These plastic odour-controlling pouches are available in many sizes, have a protective barrier applied to intact surrounding skin, and require change as infrequently as once a week. Pouches are drained as needed and are less bulky than dressings. Mobility may be facilitated with the use of these products.

## Deodorizers

Deodorizers effective in controlling biologic odours may be useful, as well as allowing cross-ventilation and fresh air into the living area. Ensuring that soiled bed linens and clothing are changed as often as possible are practical ways of achieving odour control.

## Pain control

It is essential that patients' pain is managed well both for acute episodes (e.g. around wound changes) and chronically. There is detailed discussion of this in Chapter 2.

## Summary

Care of a patient with any wound takes time. Periodic assessment of the wound is necessary, as its characteristics may change or the condition and desires of the patient may evolve. Management goals and treatment plans require review and alteration over time. Patients may present with more than one wound or more than one type of wound, adding to the complexity of management. Emotional and social issues, pain management, and management of other symptoms of the disease process are challenges that the interdisciplinary palliative care team must address. Of utmost importance, the patients and their families/care providers need our encouragement, praise, and guidance throughout the course of caring for the wound.

## References

1 Hayden, B.K. (2004). *Skin ulcerations.* CancerSourceMD.com. Available at http://www.cancersourcemd.com/tools/print/print.cfm?contentID=28316.

2 Hess, C.T. (1999). *Clinical guide: wound care*, 3rd edn. Springhouse, PA, Springhouse Corporation.

3 Haisfield-Wolfe, M.E. and Baxendale-Cox, L.M. (1999). Staging of malignant cutaneous wounds: a pilot Study. *Oncology Nursing Forum*, 26, 1055–1064.

4 Itano, J.K. and Taoka, K.N. (2005). *Core curriculum for oncology nursing*, 4th edn. St.Louis, MO, Elsevier Saunders

5 Wells, T. (2004). Palliative treatment of malignant fungating wounds. *Pennsylvania Cancer Pain Initiative Newsletter*, 39. Available at http://www.pcpi@papainrelief.org.

Chapter 5

# The assessment and management of lymphoedema

Benedict Konzen and Ki Y. Shin

## Summary

Lymphoedema is an abnormal collection of protein-rich interstitial fluid associated with chronic inflammation which leads to chronic fibrosis if left untreated. In patients with breast cancer it can cause problems which range from mild, reversible unobtrusive swelling of the arm, to gigantic and unsightly arm enlargement which is permanently disabling. Prevention and early intervention are the key to preventing this distressing condition, which is one of the most visible and intractable complications of breast cancer. Lymphoedema can develop following treatment, that is primary surgery and/or radiotherapy, or as a result of the disease from malignant infiltration and blockage of lymphatic vessels and glands. Morbidity following treatment has declined in recent years as surgery has become more limited and through the use of lower doses of radiotherapy more accurately delivered.

The prevention and treatment of lymphoedema requires commitment, persistence, and the development of new skills from the patient. In advanced breast cancer or where lymphoedema has become established the patient needs to be vigilant and exercise meticulous daily care to prevent further complications. Thus motivating and providing clear and helpful information to her is essential. This education often has to be given at a time of great emotional distress for the patient and so must be done sensitively with regular follow-up and reiteration where necessary. Many patients, however, welcome the opportunity to participate in a physical activity that can prevent complications of their treatment and disease.

In this chapter we review the pathophysiology, diagnosis (including special investigations), and treatment of lymphoedema secondary to breast cancer.

## Introduction

The practice of medicine today is complex. In the not too distant past, the physician simply took a patient's history, formulated a differential diagnosis, ordered necessary tests, and set out a care plan. With the advances in diagnostic radiology, surgical techniques, antibiotic treatment, and resuscitative measures, the general physician of today interacts with super-specialists. The doctor–patient relationship may have lost the personal touch and intimacy common in previous centuries – both the patient and the doctor have to form relationships with many different specialists to get effective treatment for one condition. The options available to us for care, where we receive care, who pays for care, and ultimately what type of care we receive and from whom is now dependent on each country's health-care system.

The palliative-care physician, hopefully, exemplifies more of the tradition of personal medical care. Careful listening and accurate documenting of a patient's symptoms should be crucial to the practice of all medical and surgical specialists. In addition, the palliative-care physician investigates the physiological disease process in the context of the psychological, social, and spiritual place of the patient. The patient is not merely a compilation of symptoms.

The patient needs to be evaluated as a whole person: the assessment needs to include her physical appearance and bearing, the symptoms from which she is suffering (such as pain, nausea, insomnia, constipation, depression), and her psychological state, both resulting from her physical problems. It is crucial to find out the patient's previous ways of managing her life, and the support network she has. The patient's condition will not be static – at any time she may be at the acute stage of presenting with, or suffering from a complication of advanced cancer, or evolving in to a more advanced stage of disease, or living with a chronic disease, or coming to the end of her life. At each stage, the palliative-care physician is called upon to assist in: disease and symptom management; educating the patient and her support network; and, finally, providing empathetic and competent care at the end of life.

To many health-care specialists, the word 'palliative' evokes an image of the dying and suffering patient – one embodiment of which is the person with cancer. Most palliative-care specialists would take exception to this very narrow view. Every sort of disease has symptoms which need to be closely evaluated and then treated.

Lymphoedema is prevalent throughout the world, with aetiologies ranging from filariasis to cancer. Lymphoedema presents one of the greatest challenges to the palliative care physician. When it reaches an advanced stage, lymphoedema is very deforming and disabling. If dealt with early, its ravages – both emotional and physical – can often be contained. The treatment of lymphoedema serves as an example of how crucial it is for medical and other clinical disciplines to collaborate if patients are to be restored physically and emotionally back to the best possible health. The successful rehabilitation of individuals with lymphoedema requires the active participation, at different times, of physical and occupational therapists, the physician, oncologist, radiologist, surgeon, and rehabilitation clinician, as well as the palliative care team. This team of clinicians must also communicate well to ensure that the patient gets the care they require from the most appropriate specialist at the most appropriate times.

## What is lymphoedema?

Lymphoedema represents an interruption in one of the homeostatic mechanisms of the body which leads to an abnormal collection of interstitial fluid. In the arm (most commonly affected in breast cancer) there will be limb swelling and, if untreated, chronic inflammation and fibrosis will follow.

## Pathophysiology

Cell metabolism depends inherently on the circulatory system. The cell requires oxygenation, nutrients, and an effective waste-removal system. The body, too, is inherently complex with multiple modes of nutrient dispersal, waste removal, and immune defence. One comprehensive organ system is the lymphatics: if this system is altered, the entire body is affected.

In this section, we will outline the foundations of the lymphatic system. From this vantage point, we will then explore how cancer—specifically, breast cancer—impacts on the lymphatic system. Treatment options will then be explored.

## What is the lymphatic system?

We often envisage the circulatory system as a fluid medium of leukocytes, erythrocytes, platelets, solutes, and proteins 'housed' in a complex network of capillaries, arterioles, veins, arteries, and the heart. By analogy, the lymphatic system is a lattice work of vessels, carrying a medium (lymph), whose purpose is largely immunodefensive. However, lymph is also involved in nourishing the living cell and removing – if not battling with – foreign antigens and waste products.

Physiologically, most of the interstitial fluid generated daily (about 18 litres) arises from the blood capillaries; 14 to 16 litres subsequently return directly, as an ultrafiltrate, to the venous circulation. The remaining 10–20%, or approximately 2 litres per day, pass from prelymphatic channels into lymphatic capillaries.[1] Lymph, the transport medium, next passes on to precollectors, lymph collectors, and then onto larger, lymphatic ducts, including the thoracic duct, before emptying into the heart via subclavian veins. Along its path, lymph is filtered through a series of approximately 600 scattered lymph nodes.[1]

With a filtration system similar to the kidney, the lymph node subserves both superficial as well as deep tissue layers. Lymph is propelled in a distal to proximal direction by surrounding arterial pulsation, muscular contraction, and ongoing respiration.

Variations in interstitial pressure allow for the transport of a protein-rich medium from prelymphatic channels, with negative pressure, to a final destination in ducts and vessels with positive pressure.[2]

Oedema occurs when there is an imbalance between filtration and reabsorption. In general, lymphoedema is the result of **venous disease**. Filtration of water is increased while macromolecules (proteins) are decreased. As the lymphatic system decompensates, water follows the oncotic pressure gradient and this leads to interstitial congestion.[3]

In contrast, gravitational oedema, as seen in a dependent or immobile limb, promotes an increased capillary filtration rate. Fluid subsequently accumulates in the interstitium. In this case, however, lymph – dependent on the propulsive effect of muscles – cannot be expelled from an already congested interstitium.[3]

## Primary lymphoedema

Lymphoedema is defined as primary or secondary. Primary lymphoedema is the result of either complete absence or hypoplasia of lymphatic vessels. It is less common and is

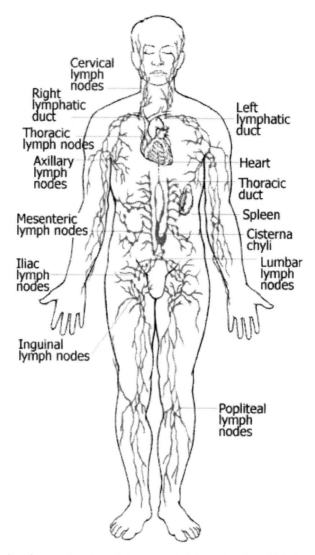

**Fig. 5.1** The lymphatic system (permission requested from Ying Guo, M.D. from her lecture *The Lymphatic System*, 2004).

further categorized into a **congenital** form (perinatal onset), **praecox** form (occurring before age 35), or **tarda** form (occurring after age 35).[4] Primary lymphoedema will not be discussed further.

## Secondary lymphoedema

Lymphoedema which occurs as a consequence of breast cancer or its treatment is secondary lymphoedema. Secondary lymphoedema is associated with many different conditions, but the end result is the interruption of lymphatic flow. Conditions leading to secondary oedema include filiariasis, malignancy, surgery, radiation, infection, and trauma.[4]

## Staging of lymphoedema

The diagnosis of lymphoedema is primarily made on clinical examination. The staging of lymphoedema is generally based on a three-stage scale – however, there is an increasing number of authorities who recognize **Stage 0** (Table 5.1). At this stage, swelling is not evident, despite alteration in lymph transport. In **Stage I**, there is an early accumulation of a high protein-laden fluid (versus venous oedema) that subsides with limb elevation. Pitting of the extremity may be present. In **Stage II**, limb elevation alone rarely reduces tissue swelling and pitting is present. In late State II, fibrosis is present and there may or may not be pitting of the extremity. **Stage III** is characterized by lymphostatic elephantiasis. Pitting is absent and the trophic skin is characteristically acanthotic with warty overgrowth.[5]

## Diagnostic imaging

In palliative medicine, lymphoedema is usually diagnosed on the basis of history and examination. The investigation and/or confirmation of lymphoedema or a specific lymphatic abnormality can be undertaken with the use of **lymphangioscintigraphy** (LAS). LAS provides images of the lymphatics and lymph nodes as well as data on radiotracer (lymph) transport. It does not require dermal injection.

Other diagnostic tools used in investigating lymphangiodysplasia/ lymphoedema include MRI, CT, ultrasound, indirect lymphography (IL), and fluorescent microlymphangiography (FM). DEXA or biphotonic absorptiometry is useful in assessing the chemical component of limb swelling, that is the percentage of fat, water, and lean mass.[5]

In general, diagnostic imaging is used if the diagnosis of lymphoedema is unclear or if an underlying malignancy is suspected. In LAS (isotope lymphography, lympho- or lymphangioscintigraphy) a radioactive tracer is usually injected intradermally. Using a combination of mobile scanners integrated with computer imaging, lymphatic vessels and nodes are visualized, and lymph node uptake speed and the rate of lymph transport are measured.[6]

**Conventional** or **direct lymphography** (CL) is an invasive technique which is not used in the routine management of lymphoedema. It is required in cases of suspected

**Table 5.1** Staging of lymphoedema

| Stage | Oedema | Elevation helps | Pitting | Fibrosis | Acanthosis |
|---|---|---|---|---|---|
| 0 | − | + | − | − | − |
| I | + | + | +/− | − | − |
| II (early) | + | +/− | − | − | − |
| II (late) | + | − | +/− | + | − |
| III | + | − | − | + | + |

+ = present; − = absent

chylous reflux syndrome or thoracic duct injury. CL involves injecting a lymph collector on the foot or hand dorsum followed by serial radiographs which delineate the lymph collectors and lymph nodes. The complications of this procedure have included allergic and inflammatory reactions as well as pulmonary embolism and damage to the endothelial lining of the lymphatic vessel.[6]

**Indirect lymphography** (IL) can be used to image the smallest of lymph vessels. A water-soluble contrast medium is injected intracutaneously. The agent is absorbed into lymph capillaries and continues to flow into precollectors and collectors. Serial radiographs can demonstrate the superficial lymphatics up to a distance of 60 cm. This technique, however, cannot define individual regional lymph nodes.[6]

**Fluorescent microlymphagiography** is used largely for research purposes. A fluorescent agent is injected intracutaneously at the medial malleolus. A fluorescent microscope and camera subsequently record the diffusion of the medium over the course of the adjacent cutaneous lymph vessel plexus.[6]

**Magnetic resonance imaging** (MRI) is costly and used primarily in tumour diagnosis. **Computed tomography** (CT) is often used to identify abdominal and retroperitoneal tumours. Tissue densities are analyzed which distinguish between fatty tissue and protein-rich fluid. Venous Doppler studies allow for the non-invasive assessment of blood flow in the deep venous system – it may help to determine whether venous obstruction is causing the swelling.[6]

## Lymphoedema as the result of breast malignancy

With the advent of earlier breast cancer detection, ongoing education, and medical screenings, one would anticipate a decline in the need for lymphoedema management. However, current techniques in caring for the breast patient still rely on general surgical principles such as tumour resection (lumpectomy, mastectomy), axillary lymph node dissection for staging purposes, radiation, and chemotherapy. Surgical resection of breast, axillary, or thoracic tumours often results in the interruption of well-established routes of lymph flow. In approximately 10% of cancer patients, the onset of lymphoedema heralds local recurrence of tumour or is the result of metastases.[7] The traumatized network of lymphatics within the surgical field frequently do not allow the rerouting of the normal (premorbid) lymph flow which still passes through this region. Lymph subsequently collects and if it is not manually (via massage or decongestive technique) removed from the area, lymphoedema will form, and eventually fibrosis. Radiation therapy may also cause scarring of the delicate lymphatic vessels resulting in ineffectual lymph flow and formation of lymphoedema.

Lymphoedema can lead to mechanical dysfunction, including a compartmental syndrome, brachial plexopathy, neuropathy, frozen shoulder syndrome, adhesive capsulitis, or myofasciitis. The pain arising from these conditions, if untreated, will lead to further morbidity and, potentially, disability.

The frequency with which arm lymphoedema occurs after breast cancer therapy depends on:

1  the type of therapy treatment used for the treatment of the breast cancer;
2  the extent of local lymphatic involvement;
3  the inherent compensatory ability of the lymphatic system.

Following surgery, the incidence of arm lymphoedema depends on the *number of lymph nodes removed*, the use and total dose of radiation therapy, and a patient's weight and age. In a study by Kiel and Rademacher in 1996, even in the absence of lymph node dissection, the incidence of oedema after breast cancer treatment was 21%. With 11–15 nodes removed, oedema was present in 27%. With greater than 15 lymph nodes removed it was 44%. Radiation therapy of the chest and axilla was associated with lymphoedema in 42% of cases.[8] Breast-conserving techniques have demonstrated a reduction in the incidence of lymphoedema.[9] Post-therapeutic lymphoedema of the arm is more common in obese individuals and with increasing age. In a study by Kiel *et al.*, 22% of breast cancer patients older than 55 were shown to have an increased lymphoedema risk when compared to their younger counterparts (14%).[8] Women returning to work during their first postoperative year were also shown to have an increased occurrence of the condition.[10] The incidence of oedema occurring after more than 2 years after surgery was around 30% in patients with breast cancer.[11,12] It is hoped that with earlier detection and the use of less invasive techniques, such as sentinel lymph node status and tumour markers, extensive surgical interventions will be used less frequently and the incidence of lymphoedema reduced.

## Pathology of the lymphatics after mastectomy

Histologically, the reparative process in the traumatized lymphatic vessels after mastectomy demonstrates fibrosis and an accompanying reduction in vessel diameter. With the subsequent ligation or interruption in lymph channels and lymphadenectomy, the body attempts a regenerative process with the formation of collateral circulation. The delicate penumbra, however, is sensitive to radiation and the use of this therapy may lead to fibrosis. Non-irradiated lymph nodes develop compensatory dilated sinuses to handle lymph volume which may anatomically be associated with a lymph node hyperplasia. If the lymphatic system fails locally, protein subsequently accumulates in the interstitium. If no intervention occurs at this point, fibrosclerosis will follow along with inflammation, scarring, and loss of regional lymphatic integrity.[7] Early conservative interventions (e.g. manual decongestive techniques) implemented early can usually prevent future intractable problems.

## Symptoms in the postmastectomy patient

The patient who has had a mastectomy is likely to have a degree of postoperative swelling, pain in the region of the surgical incision, and, sometimes, neuropathic pain in the distribution of the brachial plexus. The use of physical and occupational therapies soon after surgery are essential in order to begin a programme of limb ranging and to make an early assessment of lymph mobilization. The occurrence of lymphoedema is based on the status of collateral lymph flow. In the setting of outpatient procedures or short-stay inhospital procedures, the patient may accept marginal swelling as a complication of surgery. However, when patients experience ongoing pain, limitations in arm usage, or alteration in the appearance of an extremity they are usually more willing to seek help.

If lymphoedema occurs, in 80% of cases it will present within 2 years of tumour therapy. It often presents inconspicuously as mild oedema in the hand or forearm – often in the dorsal epicondylar region.[7] Tension and heaviness in the arm is often reported, followed by pain and reduced mobility at the shoulder. Numbness and a subjective reporting of decreased strength are also common, the former may be the result of trauma to the intercostobrachial cutaneous nerve of the arm during mastectomy.[7]

Early preventative measures in the treatment of lymphoedema include a programme of routine skin inspection (for ingrown toenails, cuticle integrity, abrasions, bruising, ulcerations, impaired circulation); use of skin emoillents; and avoidance of extremes in heat and cold, including exposure to the sun. In the clinician's office or hospital setting, blood pressure measurements, venepuncture, acupuncture, or injections *should not be undertaken* on the affected side. The patient needs to be counselled on limiting excessive exercise and avoiding trauma to the affected region from clothing (brassiere, handbag straps).[7]

## Infection

One of the leading problems in the lymphoedema patient is erysipelas. This is the result of a streptococcal cellulitis. It is characterized by localized erythema, enhanced skin warmth, and, potentially, fever, nausea, and chills. Prompt treatment with intravenous antibiotic therapy followed by oral antibiotic management is mandated.[7]

Patients are advised to exercise vigilance themselves and if they note signs of infection to start an antibiotic course immediately (those with a recurrent problem may well keep a supply at home, others need to report early for medical help). Patients should also take care of their skin and ensure that other clinicians (who may not understand the significance of lymphoedema) do so as well. It is often advisable for patients to have regular appointments with a chiropodist or podiatrist to keep their feet and nails well cared for. They should also be careful with invasive dental work and antibiotic cover for such procedures should be considered.

## Physical interventions

In the early stage of lymphoedema, simple elevation of a lymphoedematous limb often reduces swelling. Later, as the lymphoedema extends into the dependent, distal portions of a limb, therapy involves the use of a low-stretch, elastic stocking or sleeve garment.[6] The use of massage (classical massage or effleurage) may be of limited benefit. Care must be taken not to be excessively vigorous as lymphatic vessels may be damaged.[6]

### Conservative decongestive therapy

The history of conservative decongestive therapy dates back to 1892 when Winiwater recommended the use of lymphatic massage and bandaging to reduce the size of the oedematous limb. In the United States, the technique was once again revisited by Stillwell in the 1950s. However, it was not until the 1970s that Foeldi would bring to the forefront the importance of skin care, avoidance of infection, the benefits of compression bandaging, and the need for remedial exercises. At the centre of his recommendations was the use of the Vodder technique of manual lymphatic drainage.[13]

Combined physical therapy (CPT), or complete/complex decongestive therapy (CDT), or complex decongestive physiotherapy (CDP) involves a two-stage treatment programme. In the first phase, emphasis is on skin care, light manual massage/manual lymph drainage, range of motion exercise, and compression with multilayered bandage-wrapping. Phase II is a continuation of learned techniques in Phase I and aims to preserve and optimize Phase I results. It consists of compression by a low-stretch elastic stocking or sleeve, skin care, continued 'remedial' exercise, and repeated light massage as needed.[6]

CPT may be use palliatively in cases of secondary lymphoedema which results from tumour obstructing lymphatics. This treatment is usually conducted in conjunction with chemoradiation aimed at tumour reduction. In the past, it was controversial whether massage and mechanical compression would promote metastasis but, in practice, the disease is already present and the goal simply is palliation of morbid swelling.[6] Massage should not be carried out when there are extensive cutaneous metastases or local infection or thrombosis.

To maintain long-term lymphoedema reduction after CPT, a prescription for a customized low stretch elastic garment is made but this is contraindicated if there is concurrent arterial disease, ulceration, or a painful postphlebitic syndrome. The compression level is individually assessed and ranges from 20 to 60 mmHg.[6]

In a study by Ko *et al.* (1998), 299 patients with both upper and lower extremity lymphoedema underwent CDP for 15.9 days. Lymphoedema reduction averaged 59.1% after upper extremity CDF and 67.7% in lower extremity treatment. When followed-up at 9 months, improvement had been maintained in 86% of patients. These individuals maintained at least 90% of the initial reduction. The incidence of infection was also decreased by approximately 50%.[13]

## Intermittent pneumatic compression

There is controversy concerning the use of intermittent pneumatic compression and diuretic management. In late Stage II lymphoedema, fibrosis occurs as the result of an inability to mobilize interstitial proteins either into the intravascular or lymphatic compartments. The ensuing interstitial inflammatory condition promotes fibrosis and scarring which would not be amenable to a pneumatic device and actually may *predispose* to additional damage of an otherwise traumatized lymphatic network.[6] Where it is used, intermittent pneumatic compression or pneumomassage is usually completed as a two-phase programme. External compression therapy is applied with a sequential gradient 'pump'. This is followed by form-fitting, low-stretch elastic stockings or sleeves which maintain oedema reduction.[6]

## The role of surgery

There is considerable uncertainly about the role of surgical intervention in the treatment of lymphoedema. There is no accepted world-wide consensus on this topic. A debulking procedure which attempts to remove excess skin and subcutaneous tissue may actually result in the removal of, or obliteration of, superficial skin lymphatics. Omental transposition, enteromesenteric bridge operations, and the implantation of substitute lymphatics have not shown long-term benefit.

Advances continue to be made in microsurgical procedures, but their outcome depends on the skill of the surgeon, the procedure undertaken, and they often require prolonged postsurgical physical therapy as part of the treatment. The patient needs to be fully educated on the intended procedure and completely committed to it and the postoperative programme – she needs to understand the risks, the possible impairment and disability, and the demands of such procedures. Close interaction on the part of the surgeon, physician, palliative-care expert, rehabilitationist, and the patient herself are essential to the patient's recovery.[6]

## Treatment assessment

Assessment of limb volume is made before, during, and after treatment. This can be accomplished via water displacement, circumferential measurement using the truncated cone formulation, or a perometer. As previously noted, lymphangioscintigraphy can functionally document lymphatic drainage. MRI or DEXA can determine volume and tissue compositional changes. Alterations in tissue composition and fluid changes can be analysed by tonometry and bio-electrical impedance. Lastly, psychosocial indices and visual analogue scales of patient's perceptions help record personal reflections of both the disease and treatment process.[6]

## Discussion

Approximately one in eight women will develop breast cancer at some point in their lifetime.[14] The current treatment of breast cancer often involves breast-conserving surgery, axillary surgery, and radiation therapy. However, such treatments may have their own implications. Foldi *et al.* described our understanding of lymphoedema as 'chaos'.[15] Whereas our understanding of its cause and effective treatment are still unfolding, the most widely accepted means of treating lymphoedema are *conservative* in nature. These include elastic wrappings and sleeve garments, external compression pumps, and physical therapy for range of motion, massage, manual lymphatic drainage, and aerobic exercises. More controversial are surgical treatments including microsurgery and even amputation.[16]

The vast majority of individuals who experience breast cancer and its sequelae are women. Studies indicate that women are often inadequately prepared for the postoperative period or informed about support services. Of greatest concern to women in one study by Woods (1993) was body image.[17] In a study by Dennis *et al.*, active women with a stable employment history and a strong social support network were more satisfied with their lymphoedema management than women who were also combating instability in the workplace, financial constraints, or precarious social supports.[18]

Carter *et al.* (1997) extrapolates further. She described women as being abandoned by the medical establishment. Common sources of distress have included the knowledge that lymphoedema has no definitive treatment. In addition, treatment centres and lymphoedema specialists are few. More disturbing, however, was the expressed view that physicians are often insensitive and possess limited knowledge of the disorder.[16]

Many of the limitations which face lymphoedema patients in the private sector of care, such as insurance, finances, and social supports, have a tendency to be exacerbated or magnified at the hospice level. If the patient has been evaluated by a lymphoedema specialist before entering hospice and care has subsequently been initiated, supportive leg and sleeve wrappings/garments can be continued as well as traditional methods of limb elevation. Conservative care needs, such as good wound care, routine cleansing of the skin, use of moisturizing agents, and avoidance of extremes in temperature or unrelieved pressure on a limb, likewise should be continued. In a non-socialized healthcare system, it would prove difficult to initiate a comprehensive lymphoedema management programme at the hospice level. This would be secondary to limited financial resources and therapists familiar with lymphoedema management techniques. In the stable hospice patient, conservative techniques once learned by a family member may add a sense of normalcy to the patient's daily routine. The patient may feel an ongoing sense of purpose and mission. However, in the critically ill patient, emphasis will probably be placed on basic symptom management (dyspnoea, pain, nausea, vomiting, constipation) while addressing end-of-life cares with the patient and support network.

The patient's family plays a pivotal role in the patient's care. With adequate social supports, the hospice patient will have a sense of purpose and belonging. Acceptance and active care of the deformed extremity, including limb ranging and mobilization when possible, by both the patient and caregiver, will help the patient to focus on living life fully despite possible immobility. Adequately controlling pain, whether musculoskeletal or neuropathic in nature, is likewise, crucial.

## Conclusion

For any patient experiencing an illness, physical and emotional challenges are present. In the case of lymphoedema, however, the implications are more profound. Lymphoedema may signal the occurrence of a cancer or it may alter the physical appearance and functioning of a person. We define ourselves in terms of our appearance and our employment. If we are limited in these pursuits, we can become psychologically distressed.

In a study by Tobin et al., patients with arm oedema experienced greater functional impairment; increased difficulty adjusting to their illness, home-life, and personal/familial relationships.[19] Likewise, the diagnosis of breast cancer, in itself, causes significant distress.[20] Tobin maintains that while breast surgery is psychologically devastating, attempts at reconstruction and use of prostheses have helped the process of mental healing and acceptance. In contrast, the openly exposed lymphoedematous limb is a constant reminder to the patient, and the community at large, that an illness is present and that the patient is physically different from the norm. As a result, the patient may lose interest in their dress or general appearance. This loss of self-esteem may also contribute to difficulties with interpersonal relationships, social activities, and intimacy.[19]

One avenue yet to be explored is the role of palliative care and rehabilitation. Santiago-Palma *et al.* describe how palliative care and rehabilitation medicine both aim to improve the cancer patient's level of functioning and comfort.[21] Indeed the goal is multifaceted – maintenance of physical function and independence, improving quality of life, and reducing the caregiver's burden of care.[21] Lymphoedema and its management test the very foundation of this belief. Physically, impaired functioning of the limb limits activity. Cosmetically, lymphoedema may be an embarrassment and a source of social isolation and depression. There may be an alteration in a person's sense of self worth, her perception of her societal contribution, and a modification in lifestyle with spouse, family, and friends. The goal of lymphoedema management is to ameliorate symptoms and improve functioning so that living can continue.

## Key points

- Lymphoedema is one of the most distressing, potentially disabling, and intractable complications of advanced breast cancer and/or its treatment.
- It is important to try and prevent (or limit the extent) of lymphoedema by carefully-administered primary treatment of breast cancer and early preventative interventions (e.g. a simple exercise programme) following surgery and radiotherapy.
- Once established, chronic inflammation and fibrosis are difficult to treat.
- The diagnosis is clinical, though further imaging may be needed to establish the underlying cause.
- Most treatment is conservative, involving massage, elastic hosiery, and meticulous attention to skin care to prevent infective complications.
- The role of more invasive methods of treatment (e.g. surgery, intermittent pneumatic compression) is controversial.

## References

1 Stanton, A. (2000). How does tissue swelling occur? The physiology and pathophysiology of interstitial fluid formation. In Twycross, R., Jenns, K., and Todd, J., eds. *Lymphoedema*, pp. 11–21. Oxford, Radcliffe Medical Press.

2 Weissleder, H. *et al.* (2001). Physiology. In Weissleder, H. and Schuchhardt, C. eds. *Lymphedema: diagnosis and therapy*, 3rd edn, pp. 25–48. Cologne, Germany, Viavital Verlag GmbH.

3 Mortimer, P.S. (1990). Management of lymphedema. *Vascular Medical Review*, 1, 1–20.

4 Board, J. and Harlow, W. (2002). Lymphoedema 2: Classification, signs, symptoms and diagnosis. *Br J Nursing*, 11, 389–395.

5 International Society of Lymphology (2004). *Consensus document of the International Society of Lymphology*, pp. 1–7. Available at http://www.u.arizona.edu/ witte/2003 consensus.htm.

6 Zuther, Joachim E. (2005). *Lymphedema management. The comprehensive guide for practitioners*, pp. 68–69. New York, Thieme.

7 Weissleder, H. *et al.* (2001). Lymphedema in tumor management. In Weissleder, H. and Schuchhardt, C. eds. *Lymphedema: diagnosis and therapy*, 3rd edn, pp. 187–213. Cologne, Germany, Viavital Verlag GmbH.

8  Kiel, K.D. and Rademacher, A.W. (1996). Early-stage breast cancer: arm edema after wide-excision and breast irradiation. *Radiology*, 198, 279–283.

9  Schunemann, H. and Willich, N. (1997). Lymphoedeme nach Mammakarzinom – eine Studie ueber 5868 Faelle. *Dtsch Med Wschr*, 122, 536–541.

10  Liljegren, G. and Holmberg, L. (1997). Arm morbidity after sector resection and axillary dissection with or without postoperative radiotherapy in breast cancer stage I. Results from a randomized trial. *Eur J Cancer*, 33, 193–199.

11  Gregl, A. (1977). Klinische und radiologische Symptomatik des Armoedems nach Mamma-karzinom. *Ztsch Lymphologie*, 1, 9–15.

12  Pfaff, A. (1988). Einseitiges sekundaeres Postmastektomie-Armlymphoedem. *Ztsch Lymphologie*, 1, 19–23.

13  Ko, D.S., Lemar, R., Klose, G., Cosimi, A.B. *et al.* (1998). Effective treatment of lymphedema of the extremities. *Arch Surg*, 133, 452–457.

14  Carter, B. (1997). *Breast cancer facts and figures*. Atlanta, American Cancer Society.

15  Foldi, E., Foldi, M., and Clodius, L. (1989). The lymphedema chaos. A lancet. *Ann Plastic Surg*, 22, 505–515.

16  Carter, B.J. (1997). Women's experiences of lymphedema. *Oncol Nurs Forum*, 24, 875–882.

17  Woods, M. (1993). Patient's perceptions of breast cancer-related lymphedema. *Eur J Cancer Care*, 2, 125–128.

18  Dennis, B. (1993). Acquired lymphedema: A chart review of nine women's responses to intervention. *Am J Occup Therapy*, 47, 891–899.

19  Tobin, M.B. *et al.* (1993). The psychological morbidity of breast cancer related arm swelling. Psychological morbidity of lymphoedema. *Cancer*, 72, 3248–3252.

20  Wirshing, M. *et al.* (1982). Psychological identification of breast cancer patients before biopsy. *J Psychosom Res*, 26, 1–10.

21  Santiago-Palma, J., Payne, R. *et al.* (2001). Palliative care and rehabilitation. *Cancer*, 92 (Suppl.), 1049–1052.

## Chapter 6

# The management of carcinomatous meningitis in advanced breast cancer

Gillian Whitfield, Christina Faull, and Helena Earl

## Introduction

### Definition

Carcinomatous meningitis (CM) (also known as meningeal carcinomatosis or lepto-meningeal metastases) is the diffuse involvement of the leptomeninges (pia and arachnoid) by infiltrating malignant cells. Tumour cells reach the leptomeninges either by direct extension from primary tumour or metastatic deposits in adjacent tissues (e.g. brain, spinal cord, vertebrae, or skull) or by haematogenous spread. Cells are then disseminated by CSF flow.

### Incidence

Breast cancer is one of the commonest causes of CM and approximately 3% of people with metastatic breast cancer who do not have parenchymal brain disease experience clinical problems related to meningeal deposits. In addition, 6% of those with brain metastases also have meningeal involvement.[1] Autopsy studies have suggested an overall incidence of about 5.6%.[2] There is concern that the incidence of CM may be increasing as newer chemotherapy treatments, particularly taxanes, achieve better control of other sites of metastatic disease, but poorly penetrate the blood–brain barrier and do not achieve therapeutic concentrations within the CSF.[3,4,5]

In breast cancers which metastasize to the meninges, there is a marked excess of primaries with lobular elements on histology. In a series from the Christie Hospital, at least 67% had primary tumours with lobular features,[6] in contrast to the histological classification of breast primaries in which under 20% are lobular cancers.

### Prognosis

The prognosis of CM from breast cancer is very poor, with a median survival of only 2–3 months in untreated patients.[6] Death is usually due to progressive neurological disease, although other systemic metastatic disease may contribute. Many patients with this devastating condition are optimally treated with best supportive and palliative care rather than 'active' treatment. In selected patients, more active treatment may be appropriate. Some patients can be stabilized for a period of time, or until systemic disease causes death, hopefully without the reoccurrence of disabling neurological complications.

## Aims of chapter

We plan to give an overview of the clinical presentation of CM, the investigations most helpful in reaching a diagnosis, and the commonly used treatments. The aim is to raise awareness of the presentation of this condition, and to give an appreciation of the sometimes arduous treatments and their possible benefits, in order that these patients may be best supported at the end of life.

## Sources of evidence

The epidemiological and oncological management evidence is derived from a few studies of fairly small numbers of patients (largest 150, most have <100). There is very little randomized evidence to define the best treatment strategy or to quantify the benefits of treatment. The symptom management evidence-base is almost entirely derived from anecdotal practice and extrapolation from areas of clinical practice that have some similarity (e.g. the management of brain metastases).

## Presentation of carcinomatous meningitis

Patients may present with cerebral, cranial nerve, or spinal signs and symptoms, or a combination of these. These may result from injury to nerves that traverse the subarachnoid space, direct tumour invasion into the brain or spinal cord, alterations in blood supply to the nervous system, or obstruction of normal cerebrospinal fluid (CSF) flow pathways. Early on, the impairments may be very subtle and only apparent on careful history and examination. Subtle changes in mood and cognitive function, in particular, may go unrecognized, at least in the absence of more overt signs and symptoms. Neurological dysfunction at multiple levels of the neuraxis is characteristic, but other causes, such as multiple parenchymal metastases and multiple sites of bony metastases (such as base of skull involvement causing cranial nerve palsies), will need to be considered.

One of the larger reported series of CM concerns 90 patients from Memorial Sloan-Kettering Cancer Centre treated during the period 1975–1980.[7] This series excluded haematological malignancies, children, and patients who appeared terminal at diagnosis because of widespread systemic disease. The primary tumours were breast (n = 46), lung (n = 23) (13 adenocarcinoma and 6 small cell carcinoma), malignant melanoma (n = 11), genitourinary (n = 5), and others (n = 5). The most common symptoms and signs in this series are summarized in Table 6.1, in decreasing order of frequency.

## Diagnosis

Diagnosis is based on a combination of:

- clinical history and examination (see Table 6.1);
- CSF findings – positive CSF cytology being the gold standard;
- CT and/or MRI findings compatible with the diagnosis.

**Table 6.1** Presenting features in carcinomatous meningitis[7]

| Spinal signs and symptoms (in 82%) | Symptoms: lower motor neuron weakness, paraesthesias, back/ neck pain, radicular pain, and bladder/ bowel dysfunction (in decreasing order of frequency) Signs: reflex asymmetry, weakness, sensory loss, straight leg raise, decreased rectal tone, and nuchal rigidity |
| --- | --- |
| Cranial nerve signs and symptoms (in 56%) | Symptoms: diplopia, hearing loss, visual loss, facial numbness Signs: III, IV, or VI palsy, facial weakness (VII), reduced hearing (VIII), optic neuropathy (II), trigeminal neuropathy (V), hypoglossal neuropathy (XII) |
| Cerebral signs and symptoms (in 50%) | Symptoms: headache, mental change, difficulty walking, and nausea/vomiting Signs: mental change, seizures (generalized or focal) and papilloedema |

As mentioned above (Table 6.1), the characteristic clinical findings are of symptoms and signs of neurological dysfunction at multiple levels of the neuraxis. Parenchymal, spinal epidural, or bony metastases should not account for these, although concomitant metastases in these locations may be present.

Clearly, the most specific CSF finding is of positive CSF cytology (malignant cells in the CSF). This may require repeated lumbar puncture. In Wasserstrom's series,[7] 54% of patients had positive cytology after the first lumbar puncture, while 84% were positive after the second. The yield from additional lumbar punctures was very low and in 9% the cytology remained persistently negative. However, when other supportive CSF findings, including high opening pressures, CSF lymphocytosis, elevated CSF protein, and low CSF glucose, were considered, only three of 90 patients had a normal first lumbar puncture.

CT and MRI are the most valuable imaging modalities. MRI imaging pre- and postgadolinium contrast is more sensitive than CT for detecting evidence of CM. Imaging findings that strongly support CM are hydrocephalus, and leptomeningeal, pachymeningeal, or subependymal enhancement.[7,8] Dural enhancement is the much more frequent pattern in CM, seen in 83% of cases.

CT or MRI imaging may allow diagnosis when CSF results are equivocal or if lumbar puncture is contraindicated. It identifies both: (i) sites of bulk disease that may be treated with radiotherapy; and (ii) patients needing shunting for hydrocephalus. In the Memorial Sloan-Kettering series, 14% of patients had to be shunted because of intractable hydrocephalus.[7]

## Assessment

Patients with CM have significant symptoms causing change in functional ability and reduction in quality of life. These will progress over weeks or months and the focus in care must therefore be on quality of life. The assessment process is the key groundwork for ensuring treatment is patient-centred. A full assessment will require input from the multidisciplinary team, including those that have responsibility for planning care in the community.

A full history and examination should identify:

- neurological deficit
- symptom burden
- psychological status
- cognitive function
- performance status
- self care and personal safety issues
- patient insight and key concerns
- patient's thoughts and desires concerning end-of-life care
- carer issues
- social care and financial assessment.

## Treatment options

Unfortunately, the evidence base for best management is small because there are no randomized studies of CM in solid tumours with adequate power and appropriate endpoints. The aims of treatment are to improve, or at least stabilize, neurological function and, if that is achieved, to prolong survival, and therefore these would be the most appropriate endpoints. However, many studies have used only surrogate markers of response, for example clearing of CSF cytology, which may not correlate with the important aims of treatment described above.

The main treatments, which may be used alone or in combination, are:

- palliative or symptomatic treatment
- radiotherapy
- chemotherapy:
  - intrathecal chemotherapy
    - via Ommaya reservoir
    - via lumbar puncture
  - systemic chemotherapy.

Symptom management is the most important component of treatment for all patients. The oncologist in consultation with the patient needs to make an early decision on whether more active treatment is to be given. The patient's prognosis and wishes will influence whether to pursue more active treatment and what form this should take. Prognostic factors are summarized in Table 6.2; patients with a more favourable prognosis may be considered for more active treatment. However, for many poor prognosis patients, symptom management will be the only appropriate

**Table 6.2** Prognostic factors in carcinomatous meningitis

| Factor | Comment |
| --- | --- |
| Performance status at presentation of meningeal disease | In the Christie series, median survival for patients with Karnofsky Performance status (KPS) $\geq$70 (independence in daily tasks) was 313 days, for those with KPS $\leq$60 was 36 days (P = 0.0002)[6] |
| Neurological deficit | An absence of serious fixed neurological deficit |
| CSF flow | Normal CSF flow scans indicate a better prognosis[9] |
| CSF characteristics | Favourable indicators are glucose greater than 2.5 mmol/l, and CSF protein <1.0 g/l[10,11] |
| Age | Over 55 years carries a worse prognosis[10] |
| Other distant metastases | Absent or responsive systemic tumour indicates a better prognosis[10,11] |
| Response to intrathecal treatment | The degree of response at 6 weeks is indicative of survival[10] |

treatment, and many others who embark on more active treatment will cease such treatment within a few weeks because of progressive disease.

## Symptom management

Table 6.1 identified the presenting features of CM and, of course, many other women will develop these problems as the illness progresses. A holistic assessment, as outlined above, will undoubtedly reveal the need for input from the breadth of the multi-disciplinary team. Prompt co-ordination of this is vital since time is short. The palliative care clinical nurse specialist may be best placed to do this.

### Psychological issues

For some patients this may be the first presentation of recurrent disease while others may have significant other tumour burden. For all patients the implication of this diagnosis is that death is certain and the prognosis is usually at best months. Patients and families obviously need support in this. Good, sensitive communication and the provision of accurate information is vital to the patient, their family, and the primary, secondary, and specialist palliative care teams.

The discussion of treatment options must be centred on quality-of-life issues with full acknowledgement that death is inevitable and any impact on prolongation of life uncertain. Consideration of side-effects and the hospital-based time required for treatment are very important.

For some patients CM has significant effects on mood and mental status. This may be because of damage directly to the brain or non-specifically due to the impact of cancer and the poor prognosis. A psychiatric assessment may be helpful especially for those with delusional features or behaviours that are harmful to themselves or others. Drug management may be important but supportive therapies are also vital.

Altered cognitive function (e.g. forgetfulness and confusion) is very hard for those patients with insight and especially hard for carers. This is likely to worsen with disease progress and frequent, planned review of its impact on the practical, safety, and psychological needs of patients and carers is vital in preventing crises and optimizing the quality of this end stage of life. It is often these features that make it difficult to continue to provide care at home. Patients may require 24-hour nursing care (which is seldom available) and carers may become too distressed to cope with confused and agitated loved ones.

## Neurological deficit

Steroids may reduce peritumour nerve and brain oedema, thus minimizing neurological deficit and reducing associated pain or headache. To minimize the significant short/medium term side-effects of thrush, myopathy, and hyperglycaemia it is best to commence with a high dose (e.g. dexamethasone 8 mg bd) for maximum impact on symptoms and then reduce, titrating the dose to symptomatic benefit. Prophylactic, oral antifungal treatment should be considered for all patients and proton pump inhibition for those with previous peptic ulcer disease, or patients taking a NSAID or anticoagulation.[12]

When steroids provide significant symptomatic control they are often continued until the terminal stages of illness and may be given by the subcutaneous route. Because of their impact on brain oedema they may, in some patients, be a life-prolonging treatment. This may need to be discussed with the patient and their family in the context of their views on end-of-life care.

Occupational and physiotherapists have a key role in helping patients maintain their independence and safety and in showing carers how to provide safe and effective care using simple and electronic mobility and other aids. Specialist teams should be involved to assist in improving communication and visual problems and in providing most effective ways for the patient to control their own environment (e.g. appropriate nurse and emergency call systems, intercom door systems, remote controls for lights, TV, curtains, bed position).

## Seizures

There is no evidence to guide choice of oral antiepileptics in patients with CM. Specific features of seizure activity may direct selection for example:

♦ focal motor seizure – oxcarbazepine
♦ complex partial seizure – sodium valproate
♦ grand mal seizures – phenytoin.

It is preferable to select an antiepileptic that has the least need for titration, potential for side-effects, and likelihood of interaction with other drugs taken by the patient. Compliance is also key and important considerations in selection of the drug are its potential to be taken once or twice daily with the fewest number of tablets or volume of liquid.

Provision should be made for management of uncontrolled seizure activity. Oral lorazepam and rectal diazepam should be pre-emptively prescribed and stored in the house. Carers should be educated about:

- the safe positioning of the patient;
- the safe use of lorazepam;
- who to call in such an emergency, especially to avoid unwanted hospital admission;
- administration of rectal diazepam (where acceptable).

When patients are unable to swallow, subcutaneous infusion of midazolam (10–60 mg/24 hr) appears to be sufficient in many patients to control seizure activity. It can also be used intravenously to manage status epilepticus.

### Other physical symptoms

It is beyond the remit of this chapter to cover the management of the plethora of potential symptoms. Readers are referred to the many general palliative care texts available (e.g. Faull, 2004).[13]

## Radiotherapy

Radiotherapy is simple for the patient, well tolerated and can provide good palliation of symptoms. Single fractions or short courses should be used. Usually, local irradiation is given to sites of bulk disease, CSF flow obstruction, or significant clinical symptomatology. Breast cancer is moderately radiosensitive and the doses needed to treat CM effectively may produce severe marrow depression if delivered to the whole neuraxis. This may prevent the radiotherapy being continued and also prevents subsequent intrathecal treatment. In addition, whole neuraxis treatment is poorly tolerated due to fatigue and nausea.

## Intrathecal treatment

Traditionally, chemotherapy for CM has been given by the intrathecal route, although evidence is emerging that intravenous treatment may be as effective.

### Drugs for intrathecal use

There are only very few cytotoxic agents which it is safe to inject intrathecally. These include:

- cytarabine – has been used mainly in haematological malignancies, probably has efficacy in breast cancer;
- methotrexate – used in haematological malignancies and solid tumours including breast cancer;
- thiotepa – rapidly transported out of the subarachnoid space, therefore theoretically less attractive;
- L-asparaginase – only used in haematological malignancies;
- a new liposomal formulation of cytarabine (Depocyte).

### Ommaya reservoir

The Ommaya reservoir is a subcutaneously implanted reservoir attached to a ventricular cannula. It can be used for the installation of intrathecal drugs, using a fine needle to access it percutaneously, and CSF can be withdrawn, although cytology from the Ommaya may be negative when lumbar puncture cytology is positive, or *vice versa*.

The reasons for using an Ommaya rather than repeated lumbar puncture for intrathecal chemotherapy include:

- to ensure that the drug is injected into the CSF (at lumbar puncture it may be injected into the subdural or epidural space);
- to ensure good distribution throughout the CSF as the drug follows the normal pathway of CSF flow (it has been shown that drug injected into the lumbar sac may never reach the ventricular system in high concentrations);[14]
- comfort – the Ommaya is placed under general anaesthetic and its use is virtually painless.

The device is placed by a neurosurgeon, and a CT scan should be performed after placement to check correct positioning. Operative morbidity varies from under 2% (mainly haemorrhage and infection), to considerably more in several series. For example in one series (n = 44), Ommaya reservoir complications included a 17% incidence of blockage and 11% incidence of intracranial haemorrhage.[15]

## CSF flow studies

Normal radioisotope CSF flow studies (using $^{99m}$Technetium-DTPA or $^{111}$Indium-DTPA) should ideally be obtained before giving intrathecal chemotherapy. In two small series by Glantz and Grossman, 61% and 70% of patients with CM were found to have CSF flow blocks either at the ventricular outlet, skull base, in the spinal canal, or over the convexities.[16,17] CSF flow block often could not have been predicted from CT or MRI appearances; although hydrocephalus made CSF flow block likely, this was present only in a minority. CSF flow blocks may account for some cases of treatment failure and excess toxicity, especially the development of periventricular leukoence-phalopathy and dementia.[16,18] It therefore appears preferable to give local radiotherapy to normalize CSF flow prior to intrathecal chemotherapy. In around half of patients with CSF flow block, normal flow will be re-established following local radiotherapy.[16,19] In the Chamberlain series of 40 patients with initial CSF flow block, normal flow was re-established in 20.[19] All patients received intrathecal chemotherapy. The median survival was 6 months in the group with normal CSF flow but only 1.75 months in the group with abnormal flow; 20% and 70% respectively died of progressive CM. On the basis of this small series therefore, intrathecal chemotherapy does not appear effective in those in whom CSF flow remains abnormal.

## An example: the Memorial Sloan-Kettering series

One of the larger early series of intrathecal treatment is that reported by Wasserstrom from Memorial Sloan-Kettering, already referred to above.[7] Radiotherapy was given initially to sites of major clinical involvement, usually 24 Gy in eight fractions over 10–14 days (four patients had no major areas of neurological dysfunction and did not receive radiotherapy). An Ommaya device was placed prior to or immediately after radiotheraphy. CSF flow studies were not performed. Intrathecal methotrexate 7 mg/$m^2$ was given twice weekly (if WBC >3.0 and platelets >100) with folinic acid rescue. Alternatively, cytarabine 30 mg/$m^2$ was used at the same frequency if methotrexate was contraindicated or ineffective. Treatment was continued until cytological improvement or evidence of clinical stability, then reduced to once weekly, and, if improvement continued, lengthened to every 2, 3, or 4 weeks. A few patients were treated for over a year.

Overall, 23% of patients improved and in 47% neurological signs or symptoms stabilized or improved during the first 4 to 6 weeks of treatment. Among breast cancer patients, 26% improved and 61% improved or stabilized. Malignant cells disappeared from the CSF in only 19 of the 82 patients (23%) whose CSF cytology was initially positive.

Median survival for the whole group was 5.8 months and for the breast cancer patients 7.2 months. The 1-year survival was 15% for the breast cancer patients; no patient with any other primary survived more than 1 year. Of the 81 patients who had died at publication, 43% had died of progressive or recurrent neurological disease, 22% of systemic disease with stable neurological function, and 20% of systemic disease but with unstable or worsening neurology. The cause of death was uncertain in 15%. Among the 18 patients with CM and no other evidence of systemic disease, median survival was 8 months, with four patients (22%) surviving to 1 year or more and two patients (11%) surviving to 2 years or more.

Significant side-effects of radiotherapy were minimal, but would include temporary hair loss. Patients who received whole brain radiotherapy received dexamethasone 4 mg qds during treatment. Side effects of placement of the Ommaya reservoir were very few, and included one infection successfully treated with antibiotics, one mis-placement and in three patients with raised intracranial pressure who were not shunted, large extradural collections of CSF which all became infected and in two cases required removal of the device.

Side-effects of the intrathecal methotrexate included nine episodes of arachnoiditis (characterized by headache, fever, sometimes stiff neck, confusion, and disorienta-tion). This did not necessarily occur on the first treatment. All cases resolved spon-taneously in 24–72 hours and no patient had a recurrence. Methotrexate leukoencephalopathy occurred in four patients after more than 6 months and cumu-lative doses averaging 140 mg methotrexate. All of these patients had also received whole-brain radiotherapy. Three of these patients had cognitive decline, the other was asymptomatic. Despite folinic acid, seven patients developed systemic toxicity, in three stomatitis and in four marrow suppression that resulted in one death from infection.

## Combination chemotherapy, liposomal cytarabine, and lumbar administration

There is no evidence for superiority of combination intrathecal chemotherapy over single agents.

Liposomal cytarabine (Depocyte) is a sustained release formulation of cytarabine. Given intrathecally in a fixed dose of 50 mg it maintains cytotoxic CSF concentrations for at least 14 days. Dexamethasone 4 mg bd is given days 1–5 to reduce the incidence of arachnoiditis, a syndrome of headache, nausea or vomiting, fever, neck or back pain, or signs of meningism, or altered level of consciousness.[20] Plasma levels of cytarabine are negligible after intrathecal administration, as the drug is rapidly deaminated outside the CNS. The risk of neutropenia and systemic drug interactions is therefore low.[20]

Depocyte is theoretically attractive, as conventional cytarabine maintains cytotoxic concentrations for less than 24 hours, and methotrexate for less than 48 hours. The less frequent administration of Depocyte (fortnightly initially) may make administration by lumbar puncture more acceptable to the patient and perhaps may allow better drug distribution via the lumbar route, before the drug is eliminated. Although the liposomal drug is much more expensive, this could avoid the complications and expense of placing an Ommaya reservoir.

In a small study (n = 28; updated to n = 35 in the European licence application) in lymphomatous meningitis in which patients were randomized to intrathecal treatment either with conventional cytarabine (initially twice weekly) or Depocyte (initially fortnightly), there was a trend to improved survival and time to neurological progression in the liposomal arm.[20,21] In the solid tumour arena, in a small (n = 61) randomized study of intrathecal treatment with either Depocyte (initially fortnightly) or methotrexate (initially twice weekly), the liposomal arm experienced a significantly greater median time to neurological progression (58 versus 30 days) with a trend to improved median survival (105 versus 78 days).[22] Depocyte gained its licence in lymphomatous meningitis on the basis that inferiority to conventional cytarabine is unlikely, while it has a more convenient schedule of administration.[20] Depocyte does not currently have a licence for CM in breast cancer or other solid tumours.

Fortnightly Depocyte administration raises the possibility of convenient intrathecal treatment by lumbar puncture without the disadvantages of needing an Ommaya reservoir. One small study (n = 16) suggests that [111]Indium-DTPA flow studies may be performed equally well via the lumbar route, although all of these patients had a block at the basal cisterns or lower, in the spinal subarachnoid space.[23] Only two patients in this study had normal CSF flow patterns, and in only one patient was the appearance of the radionuclide recorded in the ventricular system and high cerebral convexity after a very long interval (1440 minutes). This may make it practically difficult to perform the test. Pharmacokinetic studies show therapeutic levels of Depocyte in the ventricular or lumbar spaces regardless of route of administration (intraventricular or lumbar).[20,24] However, only one and three of the patients, respectively, in the above two randomized studies received treatment via lumbar puncture.[21,22]

## Conclusion

Radiation therapy to symptomatic sites and bulk disease visible on neuroimaging studies together with intrathecal chemotherapy increase the median survival of carcinomatous meningitis to 3–6 months. Survival may be more dependent on some pretreatment characteristics than on treatment type or intensity. Whether intrathecal chemotherapy improves symptoms is unclear. In some studies it has no additional benefit,[25] in another example 40% of patients had some benefit but this was only for 1 month.[11] It is possible that for patients with adequate CSF flow, the use of Depocyte with minimal side-effects and inconvenience would allow those patients who are inevitably likely to deteriorate and die rapidly to do so without resorting to Ommaya reservoir insertion.

Evidence from randomized, controlled trials is lacking; therefore a treatment must be tailored for the patient based on her wishes, her clinical status, and the prognosis guided by literature review. The aim is to provide the most workable solution to the most difficult of palliative consultation scenarios.

The oncologist, palliative, and community services will need to work together closely to give the best possible care in what may be a rapidly changing situation.

# References

1 Gonzales-Vitale, J.C.and Garcia-Bunuel, R. (1976). Menigeal carcinomatosis. *Cancer*, 37, 2906–2911.

2 Tsukada, Y., Fouad, A., Pickren, J.W., *et al.* (1983). Central nervous system metastasis from breast carcinoma. Autopsy study. *Cancer*, 52, 2349–2354.

3 Kosmas, C., Malamos, N.A., Tsavaris, N.B., *et al.* (2002). Isolated leptomeningeal carcinomatosis (carcinomatous meningitis) after taxane-induced major remission in patients with advanced breast cancer. *Oncology*, 63, 6–15.

4 Freilich, R.J., Seidman, A.D., and DeAngelis, L.M. (1995). Central nervous system progression of metastatic breast cancer in patients treated with paclitaxel. *Cancer*, 76, 232–236.

5 Crivellari, D., Pagani, O., Veronesi, A., *et al.* (2001). International Breast Cancer Study Group. High incidence of central nervous system involvement in patients with metastatic or locally advanced breast cancer treated with epirubicin and docetaxel. *Ann Oncol*, 12, 353–356.

6 Jayson, G.C., Howell, A., Harris, M., *et al.* (1994). Carcinomatous meningitis in patients with breast cancer: an aggressive disease variant. *Cancer*, 74, 3135–3141.

7 Wasserstrom, W.R., Glass, J.P., and Posner, J.B. (1982). Diagnosis and treatment of leptomeningeal metastases from solid tumors: experience with 90 patients. *Cancer*, 49, 759–772.

8 Fukui, M.B., Meltzer, C.D., Kanal, E., *et al.* (1996). MR imaging of the meninges. Part II. Neoplastic disease. *Radiology*, 201, 605–612.

9 Chamberlain, M.C. and Kormanik, P.R. (1997). Carcinomatous meningitis secondary to breast cancer: predictors of response to combined modality therapy. *J Neurooncol*, 35, 55–64.

10 Boogerd, W., Hart, A.A., van der Sande, J.J., *et al.* (1991). Meningeal carcinomatosis in breast cancer. Prognostic factors and influence of treatment. *Cancer*, 67, 1685–1695.

11 Fizazi, K., Asselain, B., Vincent-Salomon, A., *et al.* (1996). Meningeal carcinomatosis in patients with breast carcinoma. Clinical features, prognostic factors, and results of a high-dose intrathecal methotrexate regimen. *Cancer*, 77, 1315–1323.

12 Hardy, J.R., Rees, E., Ling, J., *et al.* (2001). A prospective survey of the use of dexamethasone on a palliative care unit. *Palliat Med*, 15, 3–8.

13 Faull, C., Carter, Y., Daniels, L., eds (2004). *Handbook of palliative care*, 2nd edn. Oxford, Blackwell Publishing.

14 Shapiro, W.R.,Young, D.F., and Mehta, B.M. (1975). Methotrexate: distribution in CSF after intravenous, ventricular and lumbar injections. *NEJM*, 293, 161–166.

15 Hitchins, R.N., Bell, D.R., Woods, R.L., *et al.* (1987). A prospective randomised trial of single-agent versus combination chemotherapy in meningeal carcinomatosis. *J Clin Oncol*, 5, 1655–1662.

16 Glantz, M.J., Hall, W.A., Cole, B.F., *et al.* (1995). Diagnosis, management, and survival of patients with leptomeningeal cancer based on cerebrospinal fluid-flow status. *Cancer,* 75, 2919–2931.

17 Grossman, S.A., Trump, D.L., Chen, D.C., *et al.* (1982). Cerebrospinal fluid flow abnormalities in patients with neoplastic meningitis. An evaluation using [111]indium-DTPA ventriculography. *Am J Med,* 73, 641–647.

18 Mason, W.P., Yeh, S.D., and DeAngelis, L.M. (1998). [111]Indium-diethylenetriamine pentaacetic acid cerebrospinal fluid flow studies predict distribution of intrathecally administered chemotherapy and outcome in patients with leptomeningeal metastases. *Neurology,* 50, 438–444.

19 Chamberlain, M.C. and Kormanik, P.A. (1996). Prognostic significance of [111]indium-DTPA CSF flow studies in leptomeningeal metastases. *Neurology,* 46, 1674–1677.

20 European Medicines Agency (EMEA) (2001). *Depocyte, INN-cytarabine. Scientific discussion.* Available at http://www.emea.eu.int/humandocs/ PDFs/EPAR/depocyte/126901en6.pdf.

21 Glantz, M.J., LaFollette, S., Jaeckle, K.A., *et al.* (1999). Randomised trial of a slow-release versus a standard formulation of cytarabine for the intrathecal treatment of lymphomatous meningitis. *J Clin Oncol,* 17, 3110–3116.

22 Glantz, M.J., Jaeckle, K.A., Chamberlain, M.C., *et al.* (1999). A randomised controlled trial comparing intrathecal sustained-release cytarabine (DepoCyt) to intrathecal methotrexate in patients with neoplastic meningitis from solid tumours. *Clin Cancer Res,* 5, 3394–3402.

23 Chamberlain, M.C. (1995). Spinal [111]indium-DTPA CSF flow studies in leptomeningeal metastasis. *J Neurooncol,* 25, 135–141.

24 Chamberlain, M.C., Kormanik, P., Howell, S.B., *et al.* (1995). Pharmacokinetics of intralumbar DTC-101 for the treatment of leptomeningeal metastases. *Arch Neurol,* 52, 912–917.

25 Orlando, L., Curigliano, G., Colleoni, M., *et al.* (2002). Intrathecal chemotherapy in carciomatous meningitis from breast cancer. *Anticancer Res,* 22, 3057–3059.

## Chapter 7

# The management of fatigue in breast cancer

Catherine Sweeney

## Summary

Fatigue is a common and troublesome problem in patients with advanced breast cancer. It is a complex symptom with physical, psychological, and social dimensions. There are many possible contributors to fatigue in the majority of patients with advanced breast cancer. Management therefore needs to be multidimensional and based on thorough assessment. The impact of fatigue on the patient must be evaluated, along with the severity of the symptom and possible underlying causes.

Management involves general measures, both pharmacological and non-pharmacological to reduce the impact and severity of the symptom and specific interventions aimed at treating potential underlying contributors to fatigue. There is little evidence from randomized controlled trials to inform treatment strategies but good evidence from such trials does exist for the effectiveness of correcting anaemia in certain situations.

## Introduction

Fatigue is the most common symptom in patients with advanced cancer and is the symptom that patients report as most debilitating, with the greatest impact on their quality of life. The prevalence of fatigue in patients with advanced cancer has been reported to be between 60 and 90%, depending on the diagnostic criteria used and the patient population studied.[1] Fatigue increases with advanced disease. Prevalence of fatigue in recently diagnosed breast cancer patients was found in one study to be 16% and in patients attending for treatment or follow-up (mainly stage II disease) to be 49%.[2,3]

Fatigue is a feeling of profound, sustained exhaustion occurring after usual or minimal effort, which is not relieved by rest. An unpleasant anticipatory sensation of generalized weakness is also a feature. Fatigue interferes with the ability to perform both physical and mental tasks. It affects patients, their families, and their carers.

### Sources of evidence

There are many interventions that can be used in managing fatigue in patients with advanced cancer. Some specific interventions, such as the use of erythropoietin for anaemia in patients receiving chemotherapy, have been researched in depth and are supported by more evidence than others. Evidence supporting specific treatments has been outlined in the management section. As with many symptoms in patients with advanced cancer, more research is needed to fill in gaps in the evidence on which clinical decisions are based.

# Assessment

## Causes

It is important to know all the possible causes of fatigue in this population in order to assess and manage this complex symptom effectively in an individual. This is because in most patients there will be many possible causes, each of which will need assessment and management in its own right. Table 7.1 summarizes possible contributors to fatigue in patients with advanced breast cancer. In this patient population, fatigue occurs as a result of the disease itself, the psychological consequences of having the disease, and the various treatments used (chemotherapy, radiotherapy, and surgery may all cause or exacerbate fatigue). Fatigue often coexists in these patients with a number of other symptoms that may include pain, anorexia, nausea, vomiting, dyspnoea, difficulty sleeping, anxiety, and depression. Both physical and psychological symptoms can contribute to fatigue and a recent study of women attending a breast cancer centre found that that pain, anxiety, and depression had a more important role in breast cancer-related fatigue than did cancer treatments.[3]

## Assessment of fatigue

As already mentioned, fatigue in patients with advanced breast cancer has many possible causes and it has far reaching effects on patients and their families. It is therefore important when assessing fatigue to consider it in a multidimensional manner. Figure 7.1 summarizes an approach to the assessment of fatigue in patients with advanced disease.

Sometimes, due to the symptom itself, a full assessment cannot be completed at a single meeting and may require more than one contact with the patient. The concept of frequent reassessment is also important as the severity of fatigue can fluctuate and its importance as a symptom to the patient may vary over time. In order to determine whether or not an identified factor is a major contributor to fatigue or is simply a coexisting problem, it is important to measure the intensity of fatigue before and after treating each factor. For example fatigue should be measured before and after correcting hypercalcaemia or treating anaemia. This can be done in a number of ways, one of the simplest is to use a 0 to 10 numerical scale (0 = best, 10 = worst). It is evident, if the level of fatigue does not improve after treatment of a problem, that further treatment of the problem is unlikely to result in improvement of fatigue in the future.

## Assessment tools

Fatigue is a subjective sensation and therefore patient self-assessment is considered to be the gold standard. A number of validated tools exist for the subjective assessment of fatigue (e.g. numerical and visual analogue scales, Functional Assessment of Cancer Therapy – Fatigue (FACT-F),[4] Piper Fatigue Scale (PFS),[1] and Brief Fatigue Inventory

**Table 7.1** Possible contributors to fatigue in patients with advanced breast cancer

| | |
|---|---|
| Effects of cancer | Pain |
| | Infection |
| | Anaemia |
| | Metabolic abnormalities, e.g. hypercalcaemia |
| | Hypoxia |
| | Immobility/ deconditioning |
| | Cachexia/ muscle wasting |
| | Anorexia/ nausea |
| | Autonomic insufficiency |
| Psychological issues | Depression |
| | Anxiety |
| | Adjustment disorders |
| Side-effects of drugs | Opioids |
| | Anxiolytics |
| | Hypnotics |
| | Antipsychotics |
| | Antihistamines |
| | Antiemetics |
| | Antihypertensives |
| Cancer treatment | Chemotherapy |
| | Radiotherapy |
| | Surgery |
| | Biological response modifiers, e.g. interferon |
| Other conditions | Congestive cardiac failure |
| | Renal impairment |
| | Hepatic impairment |
| | Chronic respiratory diseases |
| | Chronic fatigue syndrome |
| | Endocrine problems, e.g. hypothyroidism, Addison's disease, hypogonadism |
| | Over-exertion |

(BFI)[1]). The severity of fatigue can be simply measured using numerical or visual analogue scales; examples of these are shown in Fig. 7.2. Tools such as the FACT-F and the PFS are multidimensional and can be used in both clinical practice and in research. Multidimensional tools have the advantage of providing additional information that can be useful in the management of fatigue.

## Performance status

Performance status is commonly measured in patients attending oncology departments. Widely-used tools that can be used to assess performance status include: Edmonton Functional Assessment Tool (EFAT); Karnofsky Performance Status (KPS); and European Cooperative Oncology Group (ECOG).[1] Both ECOG and KPS

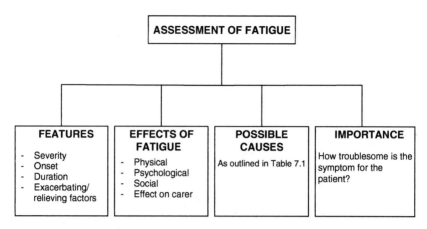

**Fig. 7.1** An approach to assessment of fatigue in patients with advanced breast cancer.

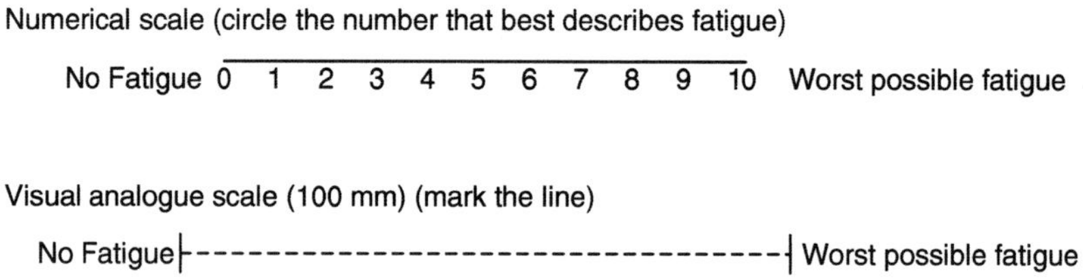

Numerical scale (circle the number that best describes fatigue)

No Fatigue  0   1   2   3   4   5   6   7   8   9   10   Worst possible fatigue

Visual analogue scale (100 mm) (mark the line)

No Fatigue |------------------------------| Worst possible fatigue

**Fig. 7.2** Examples of numerical and visual analogue scales for rating severity of fatigue.

are rated by a physician after a regular medical consultation and are widely used in the oncology outpatient setting. The EFAT is rated by a physiotherapist and, in addition to looking at the patient's functional status, it helps to identify possible obstacles to performance. These tools do not help to assess or monitor fatigue, however, as they use crude parameters to assess performance such as the amount of time the patient spends in bed. In addition, patients can be very active and also very fatigued which is not registered by assessing performance status alone. Several other tools exist that can be used in the assessment of fatigue and many quality-of-life questionnaires contain items on functional assessment. As with many symptoms, there are many assessment tools available but no single tool has been identified that suits all situations. Visual analogue and numerical rating scales provide a quick and simple way to assess severity in routine clinical practice. If further information is required and time allows, multidimensional tools or functional assessment tools may provide very useful information that can assist with developing a management approach specific to the patient's needs.

## Screening for fatigue

Fatigue is a prevalent symptom but is not always spontaneously reported by patients. Recent guidelines recommend that cancer patients are screened for the presence and severity of fatigue at initial contact and that this is regularly reassessed.[5] The guidelines suggest that mild fatigue should be followed up and that moderate and severe fatigue should be further investigated and managed as appropriate. In general, on a 0 to 10 numerical rating scale, 1–3 is considered mild, 4–6 moderate, and 7–10 severe.

## History

As fatigue is a subjective sensation, the patients self-report is of primary importance in assessment. However, very useful information can be obtained from carers and health-care professionals regarding the patient's level of functioning.

A thorough history can yield a great deal of information that may be useful in the management of an individual patient's fatigue. A multidimensional approach (Fig. 7.1) enquiring about features of the symptom, its effect on the patient and their carers, and seeking to identify possible underlying contributors is central to effective care.

Enquiries should be made about features of the symptom including severity, duration, onset, and precipitating and relieving factors. Alterations in fatigue over time may demonstrate a relationship with a particular factor (for example an increase following growth in tumour size, a change of medication, or a reduction in haemo-globin concentration). This temporal pattern underlines the importance of continu-ous assessment and monitoring of fatigue. The impact of fatigue for the patient in terms of physical functioning, social interaction, and psychological sequelae should also be assessed.

As fatigue is a very common feature of depression it is important to enquire about other features of depression (including depressed mood, anhedonia, loss of interest, guilt, suicidal ideation, poor self esteem, diurnal variation in mood, etc.) in patients with fatigue[6]. In addition to assessing for depression, it is important to enquire about anxiety and psychological distress. Family concerns are often a great burden in this patient population, particularly in patients who have dependant children

Other possible contributors to fatigue (Table 7.1) should be considered when taking a history. A collateral history from the patient's carer(s) is important in evaluating the patient's level of functioning and in assessing the carer's needs.

In addition to assessing the effects and potential causes of fatigue, it is important to assess how much the symptom is troubling a patient at the time. Sometimes fatigue is not a priority for the patient initially, due to the severity of another symptom such as pain or vomiting, but as other symptoms come under control fatigue may become more bothersome to the patient. Ongoing assessment of the patient's symptom priorities is therefore of great importance.

## Examination

A general physical examination should be performed to look for signs that might indicate the presence of conditions contributing to fatigue, such as anaemia, infection, congestive cardiac failure, endocrine abnormalities, etc. Evidence of weight loss and muscle wasting are often apparent on examination. In addition, signs of medication side-effects, for example opioid toxicity (sedation, confusion, myoclonus) should be recorded. Hypercalcaemia can also manifest as sedation and confusion and should always be considered as a possible cause of fatigue in this patient population. For these reasons assessment of cognitive function should be undertaken as part of the patient's examination. Tools such as the Abbreviated Mental Test Score (MTS)[7] or Mini Mental State Examination (MMSE)[8] can be used as screening tools for impaired cognitive function in this population.

## Investigations

Investigation of fatigue in patients with advanced breast cancer includes measurement of full blood count, urea, and electrolytes, calcium, and albumin. Blood glucose estimation may be appropriate and is especially important in patients who are taking corticosteroids. Hepatic and/or renal function tests may be indicated if impairment is suspected. If there is clinical suspicion of a possible endocrine abnormality, such as hypothyroidism, appropriate blood tests such as thyroid function tests will be required. Radiological investigations, as indicated by history and examination, should be considered.

## Assessment by other team members

Assessments by a physiotherapist and occupational therapist can provide very useful information in assessing the impact of fatigue for patient and their carer and the input of these professionals can be very valuable in management of the problem. Assessment by a psychiatrist or psychologist can be helpful in assessing for psychiatric and psychological problems that may benefit from specific treatment. In particular, a diagnosis of depression may be difficult to make in patients with advanced cancer, as symptoms such as fatigue, anorexia, sleep disturbance, and weight loss are all common in patients with cancer. In addition, patients often have worries regarding family issues such as child care, how the family will manage after their death, etc.

## Management

In planning an approach for the management of fatigue in an individual patient it can be helpful to answer the questions outlined in Table 7.2.

When fatigue has been adequately assessed its effect on, and its importance for, the patient should be known and it may be possible to identify a number of potential factors contributing to the symptom. In some patients there will be no identified reversible causes and even if a reversible cause is found for an individual patient, it is likely that there are other contributors present that are not reversible. A management approach must take all of these aspects into account and include consideration of

**Table 7.2** Questions providing important information for the management of fatigue in patients with advanced breast cancer

| |
|---|
| 1 How important is fatigue as a symptom for this patient at present? |
| 2 How is fatigue affecting this patient's life at present? |
| 3 What are the most likely causes of fatigue? |
| 4 Are there therapeutic measures available for this patient with reasonable cost–benefit ratio? |

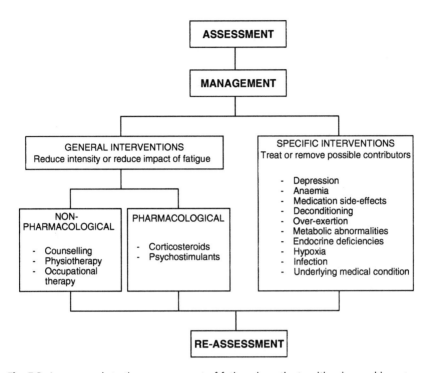

**Fig. 7.3** An approach to the management of fatigue in patients with advanced breast cancer.

general interventions to lessen the impact of fatigue and reduce the subjective sensation of fatigue, while at the same time looking at specific interventions that might correct potential causes of fatigue. Figure 7.3 summarizes this approach. General interventions include a number of effective pharmacological and non-pharmacological measures. Specific measures can also be pharmacological or non-pharmacological.

To completely eliminate fatigue is usually not a realistic objective in patients with advanced cancer and it is more practical to aim for a reduction in the intensity of fatigue and/or an improved level of functioning. Patients and their families need to be advised about what may reasonably be achieved so that their expectations of treatment are realistic. Even minor improvements can be enough to make fatigue less troublesome for the patient and to reduce its importance as a symptom.

There is evidence from randomized controlled trials that psychosocial interventions (such as psychotherapy, self-help groups) and the treatment of significant anaemia (haemoglobin less than or equal to 10 g/dl) can successfully reduce the intensity of fatigue.

## Non-pharmacological measures

### Counselling

Counselling can be very useful in allowing both patients and families to develop realistic expectations. The severity of fatigue and its impact on everyday life are often unexpected for patients and their families and as disease progresses the patient will be required to adapt to progressive limitation in physical function and activity. Counselling and informing the patient of the possible causes of fatigue and the types of therapeutic options available may allow them the opportunity to develop realistic expectations. Family members should also be given information so they can have realistic goals for the patient and be prepared for limitations in physical functioning.

Counselling of patients and their carers may allow some practical steps to be instituted to reduce the impact of fatigue. These include:

1 Adapting activities of daily living and reducing housework by avoiding unnecessary activities and enlisting help with household duties. This is may be particularly relevant for women who are mothers of very young children or teenagers.
2 Rearranging schedules within the day depending on fatigue patterns.
3 Spending more time resting or alternatively taking some exercise if deconditioning is considered to be a contributor to the fatigue.
4 Helping or encouraging patients to reduce the numbers of visitors they receive or reducing the length of visits to the patient where appropriate.

Appropriate counselling should also provide benefit to patients with adjustment disorders, depression, anxiety, and coping difficulties.

## Physiotherapy and occupational therapy

Both physiotherapists and occupational therapists can play important roles in the management of fatigue. Occupational therapists can advise on devices and appliances such as ramps, walking aids, wheelchairs, elevated toilet seats, and hospital beds to reduce energy expenditure and make mobility easier and safer for patients. Physiotherapists can also advise on issues related to mobility as well as providing passive movements to maintain flexibility and decrease painful tendon retraction in immobile patients.

## Exercise for deconditioning

It is common for patients with advanced cancer to have prolonged bed rest. This immobility results in loss of muscle mass and decreased exercise endurance leading to reduced ability to perform activities of daily living. Recent studies suggest that appropriate exercise programmes can reduce the severity of fatigue in breast cancer patients who are undergoing cancer treatment.[9] A physiotherapist can design an exercise programme appropriate to the individuals needs if deconditioning due to inactivity is considered to be an important contributor to fatigue for a particular patient. This may have both physical and psychosocial benefits.

## Rest for over-exertion

Over-exertion can also cause fatigue. It is important to consider this as a possible cause especially in younger women who may be trying to maintain pre-illness levels of activities. Rest and avoidance of unnecessary activities should be advised for such patients.

## Pharmacological measures and medical interventions

### Pharmacological treatments directed at the symptom of fatigue

**Corticosteroids** There is some evidence from randomized controlled trials to suggest that corticosteroids decrease fatigue in cancer patients.[10] Treatment with methylprednisolone at a dose of 32 mg daily was found in one double-blind, randomized, placebo-controlled study in 40 patients with advanced cancer to rapidly improve activity levels. In addition, methylprednisolone was preferred over placebo by both patients and investigators. However, the effect was short-lived and after 3 weeks of treatment activity levels had returned to baseline. The mechanism of action of corticosteroids on fatigue is unknown and it has been postulated that it may be via a mood-elevating effect on the central nervous system or inhibition of tumour-induced or host-induced substances. In addition to beneficial effects on fatigue, corticosteroids can have beneficial effects on several other symptoms that are common in patients with advanced cancer such as pain, nausea, and reduced appetite. The best corticosteroid and optimum dose has not been established. Usually benefit is seen within 72 hours of starting medication.[10] The duration of beneficial effect is limited to between 2 and 4 weeks and, in general, treatment should be tapered off and discontinued at this stage. Long-term treatment with corticosteroids should generally be avoided due to side-effects such as metabolic abnormalities, osteoporosis, muscle wasting, and immunosuppression. In considering the use of corticosteroids for treatment of fatigue, it may be helpful to weigh up the benefits of a potential 2 to 4-week improvement in fatigue with the possibility of a wide range of side-effects (including weight gain, agitation, euphoria, peptic ulceration). Often the presence or absence of other symptoms or conditions that might benefit or deteriorate with the use of corticosteroids influences the decision about whether or not a trial is warranted.

**Psychostimulants** Psychostimulants have a number of potential benefits in patients with fatigue and advanced cancer. Randomized controlled trials have found that psychostimulants are capable of antagonizing the sedating effect of opioids as compared to placebo.[1,11] In patients where opioid medication is thought to be contributing to fatigue psychostimulants may be effective. Methylphenidate has been studied more extensively than other psychostimulants in cancer patients. Methylphenidate is usually started at a dose of 5 mg twice daily (in the morning and in the middle of the day to prevent insomnia) and increased up to 10 mg twice daily if necessary after 3 days. Response tends to be rapid (within a few days) and the medication should be discontinued if a response is not seen. Modafinil, a novel psychostimulant, has been found to reduce fatigue in healthy individuals during sustained mental work and may have fewer side-effects than traditional amphetamine derivatives.[12] Disadvantages of psychostimulants include neurotoxic side-effects, possible development of tolerance, and potential for addiction.

There is recent evidence from open-label studies to suggest that methylphenidate has a beneficial effect on fatigue in the general management of fatigue in patients with advanced cancer,[13,14] although additional evidence is needed to support the routine use of psychostimulants in this more general way.

## Pharmacological treatments to correct specific contributors to fatigue

**Antidepressants** Patients with major depression should be commenced on antidepressant medication. A wide range of antidepressants is available and the choice depends on other factors. Selective serotonin reuptake inhibitors (SSRIs) are commonly used and have fewer side-effects than tricyclic antidepressants, however they can cause nausea and anxiety on initiation. In patients with problematic insomnia as part of their depression, an agent such as a tricyclic antidepressant (e.g. amitriptyline) that causes sedation may be preferred. Venlafaxine, a serotonin and noradrenergic reuptake inhibitor, causes fewer side-effects than amitriptyline but is much more expensive. Psychostimulants also have antidepressant effects and an advantage is the rapid response (within a few days) which can be beneficial for patients with advanced cancer whose life expectancy is short. The usual dosing regimen is as described above, however doses of up to 30 mg twice daily of methylphenidate have occasionally been used. Counselling should be routinely considered for palliative care patients with depression. In addition, patients may benefit from increased social support such as hospice day centre attendance.

**Treatment of anaemia** The management of anaemia depends on a number of factors. The underlying cause of anaemia influences the choice of treatment, as does the acuity with which anaemia develops. Severe, symptomatic anaemia (haemoglobin <8 g/dl) is usually treated with blood transfusion. Epoetin-alfa at a dose of 10 000 units three times weekly (increasing to 20 000 units three times weekly depending on response) has been found to be effective in patients receiving chemotherapy.[15]

However, treatment of anaemia is not always beneficial in reducing fatigue. A recent review of controlled clinical trials found that only studies in cancer patients with mean baseline haemoglobin concentrations of 10 g/dl or less reported significant benefits of epoetin treatment on quality of life.[16] The benefits of treating mild to moderate anaemia in cancer patients with advanced disease who are not receiving chemotherapy is unclear. It should also be noted that epoetin alfa treatment is not likely to be beneficial for patients with very advanced cancer, due to the delay of several weeks before significant increases in haemoglobin concentrations occur.

In addition to transfusion or treatment with epoetin alfa, treatment of underlying contributors to anaemia, such as iron deficiency, may be considered in an attempt to prevent the recurrence of anaemia.

**Review of medications** Medications should be reviewed regularly in all patients with fatigue and the use of non-essential medications known to contribute to sedation or fatigue should be minimized. If opioid-induced toxicity is suspected a reduction in dose or change to an alternative opioid should be considered along with treatment of other potential contributors, such as dehydration or intercurrent infection. As discussed earlier, psychostimulants can be used to treat opioid-induced sedation. A small open-label preliminary study suggests that donepezil (a centrally selective acetylcholinesterase inhibitor) may also be useful in this situation.[17]

**Treatment of underlying metabolic or endocrine abnormalities** Metabolic disorders such as hypercalcaemia, hyponatraemia, and hypokalaemia should be corrected where possible. Hypercalcaemia should be considered as a potential cause of fatigue in all patients with advanced breast cancer particularly in those with known bony metastases. Treatment of hypercalcaemia usually involves hydration and the use of a bisphosphonate infusion, such as zoledronic acid 4 mg or pamidronate 90 mg. Endocrine deficiencies such as hypothyroidism and Addison's disease require treatment with appropriate hormone replacement. If necessary specialist help should be sought.

**Treatment of infections, hypoxia, dehydration** Where appropriate, infections should be treated and factors leading to recurrent infections should be addressed. Hypoxia, if considered to be a contributing factor, should be assessed and corrected where possible. Consideration should be given to rehydration of dehydrated patients; this depends on the individual patient's wishes and on the potential benefits and problems associated with such treatment. Rehydration can be by oral, subcutaneous, or intravenous route.

**Optimized treatment of underlying medical conditions** The treatment of underlying medical conditions (e.g. chronic lung disease, congestive cardiac failure) that may be contributing to fatigue should be optimized.

**Control of other symptoms** Symptoms such as pain, dyspnoea, and nausea can exacerbate fatigue. Dyspnoea is sometimes difficult to distinguish from severe fatigue. A careful history of each symptom and effective treatment is essential.

**Cachexia and megestrol acetate** The progestational agent megestrol acetate has been found in randomized controlled trials to produce a rapid (within 10 days) improvement in fatigue and general well-being in patients with advanced cancer treated with doses of 160–480 mg/day.[18,19] Progestational agents are used in the treatment of cancer cachexia but this effect on fatigue was seen in the absence of improvement nutritional status.

Cachexia may contribute to fatigue and some agents that are being studied in the treatment of cachexia, such as thalidomide and omega-3 fatty acids, may have beneficial effects on fatigue.[20] The reasons for these possible effects are unclear but may involve inhibition of the production of factors (e.g. TNF-$\alpha$) by the tumour. However, it has not been clearly demonstrated that attempts to reverse cachexia result in significant improvement in fatigue and further research is needed to study potential beneficial effects of these agents on fatigue in cancer patients.

## Conclusions

- Fatigue is a common and troublesome symptom for patients with advanced breast cancer.
- Often there are several contributors to fatigue in any one patient; some may be reversible and some irreversible.
- It is essential for the best possible management of fatigue to correct reversible causes, such as anaemia, and to reassess after treatment to see if the intervention has made a difference to the patient's fatigue.

- Assessment involves consideration of the severity, effects on the patient's life, possible causes, and importance of the symptom. Ongoing assessment is vital as these factors may vary over time.
- Treatment usually involves a multimodal approach with general and specific pharmacological and non-pharmacological interventions.
- Counselling of the patient and family are vital so that their expectations are realistic.

## References

1 Neuenschwander, H. and Bruera, E. (1998). Asthenia. In Doyle, D., Hanks, G.W.C., and MacDonald, N., eds. *Oxford textbook of palliative care*, 2nd edn, pp. 573–581. Oxford, Oxford University Press.

2 Stone, P., Richards, M., A'Hern, R., and Hardy, J. (2000). A study to investigate the prevalence, severity and correlated of fatigue among patients with cancer in comparison with a control group of volunteers without cancer. *Ann Oncol,* 11, 561–567.

3 Haghighat, S., Akbari, M.E., Holakouei, K., Rahimi, A., and Montazeri, A. (2003). Factors predicting fatigue in breast cancer patients. *Support Care Cancer,* 11, 533–538.

4 Cella, D. (1997). The functional assessment of cancer therapy-anemia (FACT-An) scale: a new tool for the assessment of outcomes in cancer anemia and fatigue. *Seminars Hematol,* 34, 13–19.

5 Mock, V. (2001). Fatigue management: evidence and guidelines for practice. *Cancer,* 92 (Suppl.), 1699–1707.

6 Reuter, K. and Harter, M. (2004). The concepts of fatigue and depression in cancer. *Eur J Cancer Care,* 13, 127–134.

7 Katx, N.M., Agle, D.P., DePalma, R.G., and Decosse, J.J. (1972). Delirium in surgical patients under intensive care. *Arch Surg,* 104, 310–313.

8 Folstein, M.F., Folstein, S.E., and McHugh, P.R. (1975). "Mini-mental state". A practical method for grading the cognitive state of patients for the clinician. *J Psychiatric Res,* 12, 189–198.

9 Mock, V., Pickett, M., Ropka, M.E., *et al.* (2001). Fatigue and quality of life outcomes of exercise during cancer treatment. *Cancer Prac,* 9, 119–127.

10 Bruera, E., Roca, E., Cedaro, L. *et al.* (1985). Action of oral methylprednisolone in terminal cancer patients: A prospective randomized double-blind study. *Cancer Treat Rep,* 69, 751–754.

11 Bruera, E., Brenneis, C., Chadwick, S., Hanson, J., and MacDonald, R.N. (1987). Methylphenidate associated with narcotics for the treatment of cancer pain. *Cancer Treat Rep,* 71, 67–70.

12 Pigeau, R., Naitoh, P., Buguet, A., *et al.* (1995) Modafinil, d-amphetamine and placebo during 64 hours of sustained mental work. I. Effects on mood, fatigue, cognitive performance and body temperature. *J Sleep Res,* 4, 212–228.

13 Bruera, E., Driver, L., Barnes, E.A., *et al.* (2003). Patient controlled methylphenidate for the management of fatigue in patients with advanced cancer: a preliminary report. *J Clin Oncol,* 21, 4439–4443.

14 Sarnhill, N., Walsh, D., Nelson, K.A., Homsi, J., LeGrand, S., and Davis, M.P. (2001). Methylphenydate for fatigue in advanced cancer: a prospective open-label pilot study. *Am J Hosp Palliat Care,* 18, 187–192.

15 Demetri, G.D., Kris, M., Wade, J., Degos, L., and Cella, D. (1998). Quality-of-life benefit in chemotherapy patients treated with epoetin alfa is independent of disease response or tumor type: results from a prospective community oncology study. Procrit Study Group. *J Clin Oncol*, 16, 3412–3425.

16 Seidenfeld, J., Piper, M., Flamm, C. *et al.* (2001). Epoetin treatment of anemia associated with cancer therapy: a systematic review and meta-analysis of controlled clinical trials. *J Natl Cancer Inst*, 93, 1204–1214.

17 Bruera, E., Strasser, F., Shen, L., *et al.* (2003). The effect of donepezil on sedation and other symptoms in patients receiving opioids for cancer pain: a pilot study. *J Pain Symptom Manage*, 26, 1049–1054.

18 Bruera, E., Ernst, S., Hagen, N., *et al.* (1998). Effectiveness of megestrol acetate in patients with advanced cancer: a randomized, double-blind, crossover study. *Cancer Prev Control*, 2, 74–78.

19 De Conno, F., Martini, C., Zecca, E., Carraro, S., and Chacon, R. (1998). Megestrol acetate for anorexia in patients with far-advanced cancer: a double-blind controlled clinical trial. *Eur J Cancer*, 34, 1705–1709.

20 Bruera, E. and Sweeney, C. (2000). Cachexia and asthenia in cancer patients. *Lancet Oncol*, 1, 138–147.

Chapter 8

# The use of bisphosphonates in the management of advanced breast cancer

A. H. G. Paterson

## Introduction

The investigation and use of bisphosphonates in malignant bone disease in the early 1980s constituted an advance in the management of patients with bone metastases; they were first used in the treatment of hypercalcaemia. These drugs are now being studied in clinical trials for the prevention of bone metastases. There is a large body of evidence favouring their use in breast cancer for a number of clinical indications:

◆ in the management of malignant hypercalcaemia;
◆ in the treatment of pain associated with bone metastases;
◆ in the prevention of skeletal complications;
◆ in the prevention of further complications in patients already experiencing a skeletal complication from bone metastases;
◆ and in the prevention of bone metastases themselves.

This chapter will focus on evidence for their usage in the palliative care setting. By and large, although there is good evidence for their efficacy as a family of drugs, there is little comparative evidence that one bisphosphonate is significantly superior to another in the variety of clinical settings seen by an oncologist or a palliative care physician. Credible, large, comparative clinical trials are lacking; those trials that do exist are usually small, and generally show more similarities in efficacy than differences. Perceived differences may be more related to ease of administration, differing side-effect profiles, or successful marketing than to real differences in efficacy. There is accumulating evidence of some important toxicities which prescribing clinicians need to bear in mind.

## The clinical problem

Skeletal complications (skeletal pain, fracture, and hypercalcaemia) are major causes of morbidity in patients with metastatic breast cancer despite recent advances in endocrine and cytotoxic therapy. These skeletal complications arise because of progressive focal or generalized osteolysis. Osteolysis occurs because of osteoclast activation, either directly by tumour products or by products secreted by nearby host cells in response to tumour cell products.[1] Since the osteoclast plays a central role in focal or generalized osteolysis, inhibitors of osteoclast function can lead to clinically valuable palliation and, in a proportion of patients, to prevention of osteolytic destruction and its complications. It is also likely that the growth and development of bone metastases may be inhibited in some patients.

Some appendicular and axial skeletal fractures can be prevented. Vertebral fractures not only cause pain and disability, but may lead to spinal cord compression. In women, the problems of bone metastases are compounded by the propensity to osteoporosis. Women have a lower total bone mass than men and the threshold for developing fractures tends to be reached at an earlier age in women than in men. In addition, in premenopausal women with breast cancer, the increasing use of adjuvant cytotoxic chemotherapy and luteinizing hormone releasing hormone (LHRH) ayonist leads to early menopause with subsequent earlier accelerated loss of bone mass. There is further discussion of these issues in Chapter 9.

## Normal and abnormal bone remodelling

Bone remodelling is a dynamic process occurring in response to poorly understood physical and chemical forces along lines of stress.[2] Remodelling may result from initial stimulation by osteoblastic cells which are derived from bone marrow stromal cells.[3] Osteoclasts (derived from haematopoietic precursor cells) are recruited to an area of damaged or worn bone which is then broken down to form a bone resorption bay by the action of lytic substances secreted by the osteoclast. Osteoblasts then move into the bone resorption bay (Howship's lacuna), and new bone precursor substances, largely consisting of type I collagen, are laid down in layers which, over time, become mineralized. The formation of new bone following orderly resorption in the resorption cavities is termed 'coupling'. Bone remodelling normally occurs, therefore, as the result of a balance between bone destruction and new bone formation. Chronic inhibition of bone turnover by bisphosphonates in patients with normal bone density therefore may lead to a reduced quality of bone over time, and this must be born in mind by treating physicians.

When malignant cells infiltrate bone spaces, the balance of new bone formation and bone destruction is perturbed and bone remodelling and turnover become abnormal. Under these circumstances, three mechanisms contribute to abnormalities of bone remodelling.[4] The first occurs when a wave of bone resorption is initiated, usually focally, but sometimes generally, leading to increased bone turnover; loss of bone occurs because the resorption phase precedes the formation phase. A second mechanism comes into play when the normal connection between bone resorption and formation is disrupted and new bone is formed at sites other than where resorption has recently taken place and erosion cavities are never subsequently repaired. A third mechanism ('uncoupling') occurs when the amount of new bone formed in the resorption bays does not match quantitatively the amount of bone resorbed.

The pathophysiology of malignant osteopathy is complex. Carcinoma cells secrete a variety of substances, such as parathormone related protein (PTHrP), prostaglandin E, and transforming growth factors, which stimulate tumour growth by autocrine or paracrine mechanisms, but which also have stimulatory effects on osteoclast function. Most of these effects occur locally, but these substances can also be secreted into the circulation, and have a generalized effect on bone metabolism.[5] In breast cancer, PTHrP release also leads to increased proximal tubular reabsorption of $Ca^{2+}$ within the kidney, and this is an important mechanism for the appearance of hypercalcaemia in breast and other cancers.[6]

## 'Seed and soil' theories

The concept of malignant cell–matrix interaction is an old one, and hypotheses have been developed to explain the appearance of metastases at specific sites. These have been termed 'seed and soil' theories. Experiments designed to investigate the relationship between malignant cells and their surrounding tissues at sites of metastases suggest that chemical interactions form the basis of the association.[7]

The association of breast cancer with the development of bone metastases was first expressed in print by Paget in 1889 when he wrote: 'The evidence seems to be irresistible that in cancer of the breast, the bones suffer in a special way, which cannot be explained by any theory of embolism alone'.[8] The notion that there might be a local reason for the development of metastases at specific sites beyond a chance colonization following embolism was further developed by Batson, who described the connection between the vertebral venous plexus and the bone marrow spaces, hypothesizing a retrograde spread that would allow metastases from a primary prostate cancer to lodge preferentially in the lower vertebrae.[9] Once within the marrow space, metastases have a blood supply for further growth. Mundy has taken the 'seed and soil' idea one step further by adding the concept of a 'vicious cycle', with products from tumour-induced breakdown of bone leading to stimulation and further growth of malignant cells.[10]

## Bone metastases

The association of osteolytic, osteosclerotic, and mixed lytic/ sclerotic bone metastases with breast cancer is well known to clinicians. As the disease recurs and progresses, almost 70% of patients will develop bone metastases;[11] the median survival from diagnosis of bone metastases is between 18 and 20 months.[12]

## Bone pain

When malignant cells invade intertrabecular spaces, the malignant cells may form a mass to a size where secreted substances have an impact on local physiology. It is too simplistic to explain bone pain on purely mechanistic grounds by suggesting that a bone metastasis causes pain because trabecular fractures occur and bone collapses, leading to compression and distortion of the periosteum, a site known to be innervated by pain fibres. It is difficult to understand how bone pain can occur in the absence of fracture, but this seems to happen commonly. Bone marrow spaces are innervated by nociceptive C-fibres sensitive to changes in pressure, and it is probable that the malignant cells secrete pain-provoking factors such as substance P, bradykinins, prostaglandins, and other cytokines, which lead to stimulation of C-type fibres within bone. Prostaglandins may also play a role by sensitizing free nerve endings to released vasoactive amines and kinins.[13] The precise interaction between the tumour and bone microenvironment is unknown. Nociceptive nerve fibres staining for substance P have recently been identified within the trabecular bone of human vertebral bodies.[14]

## General principles of management

Although this chapter focuses on the use of bisphosphonates in the treatment of bone metastases in breast cancer, it is important to recognize that other modalities continue to provide the mainstay of therapy in most patients.

Bone pain management includes a thorough history and physical examination, full discussion with the patient about a plan of action, and attempts to modify the pathological process. These attempts include external beam radiotherapy (still the most effective remedy for alleviation of localized bone pain) and palliative chemotherapy. A good response to chemotherapy includes subjective relief of symptoms, including pain. Hormone therapy can provide a high quality remission in breast cancer patients with bone metastases.

Elevation of the pain threshold with the use of non-pharmacological methods as well as analgesics, interruption of pain pathways by local or regional anaesthesia or neurolysis, and modification of lifestyle are all helpful, but invariably opioid and other adjuvant analgesic management will be required.

Prophylactic surgery and radiation therapy for patients with cortical erosion caused by metastasis in the femur and humerus may prevent the distress of a pathological fracture.

## Bisphosphonates

Many bisphosphonates have been assessed in the management of malignant bone disease. These include etidronate, pamidronate, clodronate, residronate, mildronate, neridronate, alendronate, ibandronate, and zoledronate. Pamidronate, ibandronate, zoledronate, and clodronate have been the most extensively studied and are widely available for the treatment of malignant hypercalcaemia, Paget's disease of bone, osteoporosis, and other less common indications. Pamidronate, clodronate, zoledronate, and ibandronate all lead to an effective lowering of serum calcium which is attributable to decreased bone resorption. Pamidronate, an aminobisphosphonate, is not ideal for oral use because of dose-related gastrointestinal toxicity. There is evidence that long-term pamidronate administered orally may also induce osteomalacia[15] and this may be the case for most chronically administered bisphosphonates, whether given orally or intravenously. Clodronate is effective when given intravenously for hypercalcaemia and bone pain and can be used orally. Its long-term administration appears not to be associated with a defect in the mineralization of bone.[16]

The geminal bisphosphonates are analogues of pyrophosphate characterized by a stable P–C–P bond. They bind with high affinity to hydroxyapatite crystals in bone, and are potent inhibitors of normal and pathological bone resorption.[17] At the cellular level several mechanisms of action seem to operate, the dominant mechanism differing in different compounds, but all appear to have a final common effect of inhibition of osteoclast function. The osteoblast might be the initial target cell for bisphosphonates, exerting an effect on the osteoclast by modulation of stimulating and inhibiting factors which control osteoclast function.[18]

These agents appear to promote apoptosis in murine osteoclasts both *in vivo* and *in vitro*, the more potent bisphosphonates exhibiting the greatest apoptotic action.[19] In the absence of apoptosis, inhibition of osteoclast function appears to be mediated by osteoblasts, which produce a factor inhibiting osteoclastic function.[20] This action does not interfere with the ability of cells of the monocyte–macrophage lineage to produce colonies.[21] Bisphosphonates can also inhibit the proliferation and promote the cell death of macrophages.[22,23] Again, the process is one of apoptosis rather than necrosis and might, in part, explain the pain-relieving properties of bisphosphonates. Shipman *et al.* have described the induction of apoptosis by bisphosphonates in human myeloma cell lines.[24]

At the molecular level, bisphosphonates fall into two broad classes: nitrogen containing and non-nitrogen containing. These two groups have different molecular mechanisms of action. Nitrogen-containing bisphosphonates, such as pamidronate, alendronate, and ibandronate inhibit the mevalonate signalling pathway in osteoclasts while non-nitrogen containing bisphosphonates are incorporated into ATP forming non-hydrolysable analogues.[25] Differences in side-chain moieties account for the variation in potency between the various bisphosphonates, a feature much trumpeted by the marketing departments of some pharmaceutical companies. There is no level 1 evidence from clinical trials that these differences in potencies translate to major advantages in clinical efficacy.

## Clinical trials and use of bisphosphonates in breast cancer

### Hypercalcaemia

As a result of secretion of factors from infiltrating malignant ductal cells acting focally and humorally, osteoclast activity is markedly increased, with a reduction in osteoblast activity, leading to 'uncoupling' of bone resorption and formation.[26] Parathyroid hormone related protein (PTHrP) appears to play a central role in the malignant hypercalcaemia of breast cancer.[27]

We have reviewed the evidence for the treatment of hypercalcaemia and have offered some broad guidelines.[28] Randomized trials in hypercalcaemic patients are notoriously difficult to carry out due to the poor clinical status of most patients, the questionable ethics of a non-treated control group, the difficulty in obtaining satisfactory consent, and the widely variable response rate which depends on the underlying primary malignancy. For example the hypercalcaemia of myeloma responds more easily to treatment than the hypercalcaemia associated with carcinoma of the lung. Saline rehydration will usually effect a median reduction of 0.25 mM/l but its effect is transient.[29] Rehydration is useful for treating mild degrees of hypercalcaemia but usually should be accompanied by bisphosphonate therapy. Symptomatic hypercalcaemia, especially with levels of $Ca^{2+}$ greater than 3.0 mM/l, requires vigorous rehydration (N-saline 150–200 ml/h with KCl 20–40 mEq/l added), and the administration of clodronate 1500 mg in 500 ml physiological saline over 2 h, or pamidronate 60–90 mg in 250–500 ml physiological saline over 2 h, or zoledronate 4 mgms iv over 15 min. Pamidronate may give a longer duration of maintenance of normocalcaemia[30] than clodronate (28 days median vs. 14 days) but in many countries is significantly more expensive. Newer bisphosphonates, such as ibandronate and zoledronate, are currently being studied. Ibandronate at doses of 4–6 mg iv and zoledronate at 4 mg iv appear to be at least as efficacious as pamidronate.[31,32] Although it is more expensive, it has been suggested that zoledronate may be superior to pamidronate with a higher rare of response and longer duration of response, and with the added advantage of a shorter infusion time. These studies are difficult to assess, since results are heavily dependent on the clinical case mix and are of low power, often relying on pooling of trials results (level 2 evidence). Clodronate can be safely and effectively given subcutaneously, normalizing the serum calcium within 5 days in 32 of 43 infusions given in a palliative care unit.[33] Many units use specially prepared baby bottles with balloon bags containing 240 ml of normal saline into which the bisphosphonate can be injected in the pharmacy for outpatient delivery of pamidronate or clodronate. The balloons can be prepared so that delivery rates of around 100 ml/h are achieved.

## Reduction of skeletal complications

Early clinical investigations of bisphosphonates were carried out in uncontrolled trials of patients with advanced disease or small non-placebo controlled, open studies.[34] Although these investigators were probably correct in their conclusions, it is difficult to determine the extent to which patient selection and the placebo effect influenced the positive results of the investigations.

One of the first randomized, controlled studies to be published was an open trial of the aminobisphosphonate, pamidronate, given orally for 2 years at 300 mg daily in patients with bone metastases from breast cancer.[35] The investigators demonstrated a reduction in the skeletal complications of hypercalcaemia and vertebral fractures. Radiation treatments for bone pain were also reduced, but there was difficulty in patient compliance due to a high rate of upper gastrointestinal side-effects (level 2 evidence).

In a double-blind, randomized, placebo-controlled trial of oral clodronate, 1600 mg given daily for 2 years, we confirmed this beneficial effect on skeletal morbidity in patients with bone metastases from breast cancer.[36] The number of patients suffering from episodes of hypercalcaemia and the total number of episodes were reduced; the number of major vertebral fractures and the vertebral deformity rate were also reduced; and the number of radiation therapy treatments was lower in the clodronate-treated patients. No survival benefit was evident (level 1 evidence). McCloskey et al. reviewed the pre-entry and follow-up vertebral fracture prevalence in 163 of the 173 patients in this trial and found that 46% of the patients had evidence of vertebral fracture at trial entry.[37] The patients deriving the greatest benefit from the oral clodronate were those who had already sustained vertebral fractures and were therefore at greatest risk for sustaining further fractures. This trial enrolled patients with more advanced bone disease and was smaller than later trials of pamidronate and zoledronate.

Pamidronate, which can occasionally induce sclerosis in osteolytic lesions when used as the only therapy,[38] has been investigated in several trials. Measurement of response in bone is a difficult process and unless differences in the arms of a trial are large, small but significant differences can be missed. Tumour response in bone and duration of response were assessed in a double-blind, randomized trial, which showed similar response rates in bone but a significantly ($p = 0.02$) increased duration of response for patients receiving pamidronate 45 mg given intravenously every 3 weeks (249 days median time to progression compared to 168 days in controls).[39] Theriault *et al.* have reported a randomized trial of 380 patients with recurrent breast cancer in bone and demonstrated a convincing reduction in the skeletal complications of vertebral fracture, pain, and hypercalcaemia with intravenous pamidronate 90 mg given monthly for 2 years.[40] No survival benefit was apparent. A trial of intravenous pamidronate in 372 patients with bone metastases from carcinoma of the breast receiving hormone therapy has shown a similar reduction in skeletal complications.[41]

Zoledronate has been assessed in comparison to pamidronate in patients with breast cancer and myeloma. Median time to first event was similar for both agents.[42] Using an Anderson–Gill statistical model (which also accounts for the frequency of events subsequent to the first event) it has been suggested that zoledronate was the superior agent. The increased costs of zoledronate in the absence of a survival benefit or clear-cut quality of life benefit have led us to take a decision not to fund this agent for the prevention of bone metastases in breast cancer.

As a result of these trials giving level 1, grade A evidence, we currently recommend the use of either oral clodronate 1600 mg orally daily (preferably taken one-half hour to 1 hour before breakfast or at least 2 hours away from food) or intravenous pamidronate 90 mg every 4 weeks in patients with radiologically established bone metastases from breast cancer. While the use of bisphosphonates to prevent skeletal complications is an advance, it must be stated that the cost (especially the cost of the high potency agents which are still on patent) to prevent one skeletal complication is very high and is at the limits of what some individuals and societies would say was really worthwhile. The cost of avoiding one skeletal complication in prostate cancer patients with zoledronate is over US $100 000.[43] In breast cancer the figure seems to be lower with pamidronate coming in at around US $75 000 per quality adjusted life year.

A common clinical question raised is how long should one continue bisphosphonate therapy. There are no clinical studies to guide the clinician here. It is our practice to continue treatment for as long as the patient has symptoms requiring treatment. There is little evidence that true resistance develops and the practice of changing bisphosphonates (e.g. from clodronate to pamidronate or *vice versa*) on progression of disease has little backing in clinical research. It is more likely that tumour burden has increased to the level that bone turnover is accelerated – increasing the dosage may produce reduction in the accelerated turnover.

## Bone pain

The notion that bisphosphonates might decrease bone pain in some patients with bone metastases arose from clinical observations of patients receiving bisphosphonates for hypercalcaemia. Patients experienced not only normalization of serum $Ca^{2+}$ and relief of the symptoms of hypercalcaemia, but also reported relief of pain.

Ernst *et al.* demonstrated, in a double-blind, cross-over trial of intravenous clodronate in patients with bone pain caused by a variety of malignancies, that clodronate had useful analgesic properties (level 2 evidence).[44] This was confirmed (level 1 evidence) in a larger randomized, double-blind, controlled trial of intravenous clodronate in patients with metastatic bone pain.[45] No dose–response relationship was seen. Improvement in pain and mobility scores had been described in a previously reported trial of oral pamidronate, although these patients had not been selected specifically because of bone pain but because they had osteolytic metastases.[46] However, the modest effect, coupled with its poor oral tolerability as demonstrated by Coleman *et al.*,[47] make oral pamidronate unlikely to supersede its intravenous counterpart. Level 1 evidence of pain relief has also been described with intravenous pamidronate in the previously discussed placebo-controlled trial in patients with bone metastases from breast cancer.[48] The mechanism of pain relief is unknown but may be related to osteoclast and macrophage apoptosis or an inhibition of pain-provoking cytokines.

Ibandronate, a potent nitrogen-containing bisphosphonate, has been shown to reduce skeletal complications of metastatic breast cancer but has also demonstrated significant and lasting pain relief and improved quality of life when given intravenously at a dose of 6 μg repeated monthly in patients with bone metastases from metastatic breast cancer.[49] The drug is also efficacious in reducing the risk of skeletal complications in metastatic breast cancer when used orally and seems to be well tolerated at doses of 50 μg daily.[50]

## Some problems

Bone turnover is a normal repair mechanism and basic multicellular units (bone resorption bays) are formed in order to repair areas of effete or damaged bone. Bisphosphonates are potent inhibitors of bone turnover and therefore it is not surprising that the quality of bone formed when long-term potent bisphosphonates are used in patients with non-osteoporotic bone may be inferior to normal bone. Recently, 63 cases of osteonecrosis of the maxilla and mandible have been reported in patients receiving intravenous pamidronate and zoledronate (55 patients) and oral risedronate and alendronate (8 patients).[51] This is a painful, non-healing necrosis of the tooth socket following dental extraction leading to osteonecrosis of the mandible or maxilla. It is an extremely difficult condition to treat, usually requiring major excision of bone. The pathological changes seen are similar to those seen with severe radiation necrosis. Bisphosphonates certainly have the potential for interference with mineralization and healing. Their half-life is several years. Increased fractures have been observed in Paget's disease with etidronate[52] and a case report of osteopetrosis in a child on iv pamidronate which also led to increased fractures[53] indicates that these agents must be used with care, using the lowest dose and frequency which is efficacious for the end-point sought. Their routine use for months (and sometimes years) on end with minimum supervision is poor practice.

# Conclusions

The following suggestions are submitted for consideration by physicians treating patients with breast cancer:

- Malignant hypercalcaemia: intravenous pamidronate, clodronate, ibandronate or zoledronate with rehydration as described in the text (level 3, grade A evidence). Newer, more potent drugs, such as ibandronate or zoledronate, may offer some advantages with shorter infusion times, but are significantly more expensive. Clodronate can also be given subcutaneously. In some countries (Australia and Canada for example), it is routine for palliative care teams to give these drugs at home. This makes life for the patient easier and also reduces time and space needed on day therapy units.
- Presence of bone metastases (symptomatic or asymptomatic): oral clodronate 1600 mg orally daily (taken one-half hour to 1 hour before breakfast) or pamidronate 90 mg every 4 weeks iv (level 1, grade A evidence). Zoledronate 4 mgms iv or ibandronate 6 mgms iv is at least as effective as pamidronate but is significantly more expensive.
- Moderate to severe bone pain: pamidronate 90 mg intravenously every 4 weeks; clodronate 1500 mg iv every 2–3 weeks (level 1, grade A evidence). Ibandronate 6 mgms iv is an interesting addition and may have particularly useful analgesic properties. Clinical trials are underway.

# References

1 Mundy, G.R., Ibbotson, K.J., DeSouza, S.M. *et al.* (1984). The hypercalcemia of cancer. Clinical Implication and pathogenic mechanisms. *N Eng J Med*, **310**, 1718–1727.

2 Kaplan, F.S. (1987). Osteoporosis: pathophysiology and prevention. *Clinical symposia No 4.* Ciba-Geigy.

3 Mundy, G.R. (1987). Bone resorption and turnover in health and disease. *Bone*, **8** (Suppl. 1), S9–16.

4 Kanis, J.A. and McCloskey, E.V. (1997). Bone turnover and biochemical markers in malignancy. *Cancer*, **80** (Suppl 8), 1538–1545.

5 Mundy, G.R. (1988). Hypercalcemia of malignancy revisited. *J Clin Invest*, **82**, 1–6.

6 Kanis, J.A., Percival, R.C., Yates, A.J.P., *et al.* (1986). Effects of diphosphonates in hypercalcemia due to neoplasia. *Lancet*, I, 615–616.

7 Kamenor, B., Kieran, M.W., Barrington-Leigh, J., *et al.* (1984). Homing receptors as functional markers for classification, prognosis, and therapy of leukemia and lymphomas. *Proceed Soc Exp Biol Med*, **177**, 211–219.

8 Paget, S. (1889). The distribution of secondary growths in cancer of the breast. *Lancet*, I, 571–573.

9 Batson, O.V. (1940). The function of the vertebral veins and their role in the spread of metastases. *Ann Surg*, **112**, 138.

10 Mundy, G.R. (1997). Mechanisms of bone metastasis. *Cancer*, **80** (Suppl 8), 1546.

11 Coleman, R.E. and Rubens, R.D. (1987). The clinical course of bone metastases from breast cancer. *Br J Cancer*, **55**, 61–66.

12 Paterson, A.H.G. (1987). Natural history of skeletal complications of breast cancer, prostate cancer and myeloma. *Bone*, 8 (Suppl. 1), S17–S22.

13 Ferreira, S.H. (1983). Prostaglandins: peripheral and central analgesia. *Adv Pain Res Therapy*, 5, 627–634.

14 Fras, C., Kravetz, P., Mody, D.R., and Heggeness, M.H. (2003). Substance P-containing nerves within the human vertebral body: an immunohistochemical study of the basivertebral nerve. *Spine J*, 3, 63–67.

15 Adamson, B.B., Gallacher, S.J., Byars, J., *et al.* (1993). Mineralization defects with pamidronate therapy for Paget's disease. *Lancet*, 342, 1459–1460.

16 Taube, T., Elomaa, I., Blomqvist, C., *et al.* (1993). Comparative effects of clodronate and calcitonin in metastatic breast cancer. *Eur J Clin Oncol*, 29, 1677–1681.

17 Fleisch, H. (2000). *Bisphosphonates in bone disease – from the laboratory to the patient*, 4th edn. San Diego and London, Academic Press.

18 Sahni, M., Guenther, H.L., Fleisch, H., *et al.* (1993). Bisphosphonates act on rat bone resorption through the mediation of osteoblasts. *J Clin Invest*, 91, 2004–2011.

19 Hughes, D.E., Wright, K.R., Uy, H.L., *et al.* (1995). Bisphosphonates promote apoptosis in murine osteoclasts *in vitro* and *in vivo*. *J Bone Mineral Res*, 10, 1478–1487.

20 Siwec, B., Lacroix, M., DePllak, C., *et al.* (1997). Secretory products of breast cancer cells specifically affect human osteoblastic cells: partial characterization of active factors. *J Bone Mineral Res*, 12, 552–560.

21 Nishikawa, M., Akatsu, T., and Katayama, Y. (1996). Bisphosphonates act on osteoblastic cells and inhibit osteoclast formation in mouse marrow cultures. *Bone*, 18, 9–14.

22 Selander, K.S., Monkkonen, J., Karhukorpi, E.K., *et al.* (1996). Characteristics of clodronate-induced apoptosis in osteoclasts and macrophages. *Mol Pharmacol*, 50, 1127–1138.

23 Rogers, M.J., Chilton, K.M., Coxon, F.P., *et al.* (1996). Bisphosphonates induce apoptosis in mouse macrophage-like cells in vitro by a nitric oxide independent mechanism. *J Bone Mineral Res*, 11, 1482–1491.

24 Shipman, C.M., Rogers, M.J., Apperley, J.F., *et al.* (1997). Bisphosphonates induce apoptosis in human myeloma cell lines: a novel anti-tumour activity. *Br J Haematol*, 98, 665–672.

25 Rogers, M.J., Gordon, S., Benford, H.L., *et al.* (2000). Cellular and molecular mechanisms of action of bisphosphonates. *Cancer*, 88 (S12), 2961–2978.

26 Body, J.J. and Delmas, P.D. (1992). Urinary pyridinium cross-links as markers of bone resorption in tumour-associate hypercalcemia. *J Clin Endocrinol Metabol*, 74, 471–475.

27 Grill, V., Ho, P., Body, J.J., *et al.* (1991). Parathyroid hormone-related protein: elevated levels in both humoral hypercalcemia of malignancy and hypercalcemia complicating metastatic breast cancer. *J Clin Endocrinol Metabol*, 73, 1309–1315.

28 Body, J.J., Bartl, R., Burckhardt, P., *et al.* (1998) Current use of bisphosphonates in oncology. International Bone and Cancer Study Group. *J Clin Oncol*, 16, 3890–3899.

29 Singer, F.R., Rich, P.S., Lad, T.E., *et al.* for the Hypercalcemia Study Group (1991). Treatment of hypercalcemia of malignancy with intravenous etidronate. A controlled, multicenter study. *Arch Int Med*, 151, 471–476.

30 Purohit, O.P., Radstone, C.R., Anthony, C., *et al.* (1995). A randomised double-blind comparison of intravenous pamidronate and clodronate in the hypercalcemia of malignancy. *Br J Cancer*, 71, 1289–1293.

31 Ralston, S.H., Thiebaud, D., Hermann, Z., *et al.* (1997). Dose response study of ibandronate in the treatment of cancer associated hypercalcemia. *Br J Cancer*, 75, 295–300.

32 Major, P., Lortholary, A., and Hon, J. (2001). Zoledronic acid is superior to pamidronate in the treatment of hypercalcemia of malignancy: a pooled analysis of two randomized, controlled trials. *J Clin Oncol*, 19, 558–567.

33 Roemer-Becuwe, C., Vigano, A., Romano, F., *et al.* (2003). Safety of subcutaneous clodronate and efficacy in hypercalcemia of malignancy: a novel route of administration. *J Pain Symptom Manage*, 26, 843–848.

34 Elomaa, I., Blomqvist, C., Porrka, L., *et al.* (1987). Treatment of skeletal disease in breast cancer: a controlled clinical trial. *Bone*, 8 (Suppl. 1), S53–S56.

35 van Holten Verzanvoort, A.T., Bijvoet, O.L., Cleton, F.J., *et al.* (1987). Reduced morbidity from skeletal metastases in breast cancer patients during long-term bisphosphonates (APD) treatment. *Lancet*, 11, 983–985.

36 Paterson, A.H.G., Powles, T.J., Kanis, J.A., *et al.* (1993). Double-blind controlled trial of oral clodronate in patients with bone metastases from breast cancer. *J Clin Oncol*, 11, 59–65.

37 McCloskey, E.V., Spector, T.D., Eyres, K.S., *et al.* (1993). The assessment of vertebral deformity: a method for use in population studies and clinical trials. *Osteoporosis Internat*, 3, 138–147.

38 Coleman, R.E., Woll, P.J., Miles, M., *et al.* (1988). Treatment of bone metastases from breast cancer with (3-amino-1-hydroxy- propylidene)-1, 1-bisphosphonate (APD). *Br J Cancer*, 58, 621–625.

39 Conte, P.F., Latreille, J., Mauriac, L., *et al.* (1996). Delay in progression of bone metastases in breast cancer patients treated with intravenous pamidronate: results from a multinational randomised controlled trial. *J Clin Oncol*, 14, 2552–2559.

40 Hortobagyi, G.N., Theriault, R.L., Porter, L., *et al.* (1996). Efficacy of pamidronate in reducing skeletal complications in patients with breast cancer and lytic bone metastases. *N Eng J Med*, 335, 1785–1791.

41 Theriault, R.L., Lipton, A., Hortobagy, G.N., *et al.* (1999). Pamidronate reduces skeletal morbidity in women with advanced breast cancer and lytic bone lesions: a randomized placebo controlled trial. *J Clin Oncol*, 17, 846–854.

42 Rosen, L.S., Gordon, D., Kaminski, M., *et al.* (2001). Zoledronic acid versus pamidronate in the treatment of skeletal metastases in patients with breast cancer or osteolytic lesions of multiple myeloma: a phase III, double-blind, comparative trial. *Cancer J*, 7, 377–387.

43 Reed, S.D., Radeva, J.I., Glendinning, G.A., Saad, F., and Schulman, K.A. (2004). Cost-effectiveness of zoledronic acid for the prevention of skeletal complications in patients with prostate cancer. *J Urol*, 171, 1537–1542.

44 Ernst, D.S., MacDonald, N., Paterson, A.H.G., *et al.* (1992). A double-blind cross-over trial of intravenous clodronate in metastatic bone pain. *J Pain Symptom Manage*, 7, 4–11.

45 Ernst, D.S., Brasher, P., Hagen, N.A., *et al.* (1997). A randomised, controlled trial of intravenous clodronate in patients with metastatic bone disease and pain. *J Pain Symptom Manage*, 13, 319–326.

46 van Holten Verzanvoort, A.T., Zwinderman, A.H., Aaranson, N.K., *et al.* (1991). The effect of supportive pamidronate treatment on aspects of quality of life of patients with advanced breast cancer. *Eur J Cancer*, 27, 544–549.

47 Coleman, R.E., Houston, S., Purohit, O.P., *et al.* (1998). A randomized Phase II evaluation of oral pamidronate for advanced bone metastases from breast cancer. *Eur J Cancer*, 34, 820–824.

48 Hortobagyi, G.N., Theriault, R.L., Porter, L., *et al.* (1996). Efficacy of pamidronate in reducing skeletal complications in patients with breast cancer and lytic bone metastases. *N Eng J Med*, 335, 1785–1791.

49 Diel, I.J., Body, J.J., Lichinister, M.R., *et al.* (2004). Improved quality of life after long-term treatment with the bisphosphonate ibandronate in patients with metastatic bone disease due to breast cancer. *Eur J Cancer*, 40, 1704–1712.

50 Body, J.J., Diel, I.J., Lichinitzer, M.R., *et al.* (2004). Oral ibandronate reduces the risk of skeletal complications in breast cancer patients with metastatic bone disease: results from two randomized, placebo-controlled Phase 3 studies. *Br J Cancer*, 90, 1133–1137.

51 Ruggiero, S.L., Mehrotra, B., Rosenberg, T.J., and Engroff, S.L. (2004). Osteonecrosis of the jaws associated with the use of bisphosphonates: a review of 63 cases. *J Oral Maxillofac Surg*, 62, 527–534.

52 Eyres, K.S., Marshall, P., McCloskey, E.V., Douglas, D.L., and Kanis, J.A. (1992). Spontaneous fractures in a patient treated with low doses of etidronic acid (disodium etidronate). *Drug Saf*, 7, 162–165.

53 Whyte, M.P., Wenkert, D., Clements, K.L., *et al.* (2003). Bisphosphonate-induced osteopetrosis. *N Engl J Med*, 349, 457–463.

Chapter 9

# The management of pain and other complications from bone metastases

Yolanda Zuriarrain Reyna and Eduardo Bruera

## Introduction

Breast cancer is the most common cancer in women and one of the most feared. With recent advances in treatment its mortality is falling and women are living longer with a chronic disease – some are symptom-free and others may have significant morbidity or be symptomatic intermittently. It is important to design a treatment strategy for every stage of the disease. Staging procedures should follow algorithms that focus on assessment of prognosis and specific therapeutic possibilities for operable and advanced disease.

The incidence of breast cancer is increasing in many industrialized countries and is a major health problem, with 1 million new cases diagnosed annually worldwide.[1] In the US, it is the most frequently diagnosed cancer in women and accounts for 30% of all cancers diagnosed and 16% of all cancer deaths in women.[2] The incidence rate rises steadily up to the age of 50 years. In postmenopausal women the rate of increase slows down, although the incidence continues to rise at a mean rate of 0.8–3% annually in many European countries. Mortality rates for breast cancer in Europe and North America are in the order of 18–23 per 100 000 women, with an incidence rate of 62– 100 per 100 000 women.[3]

Geographical variations of incidence are well known and extensively described, with the highest rates in Western countries (100 cases/ 100 000 women) and lowest rates in Asian countries (15–20 cases/ 100 000 women).[2,3,4]

In about 10% of patients breast cancer is diagnosed at the stage of overt, advanced disease; it is one of the most common causes of bone metastases. About 65–75% of patients with advanced breast cancer suffer from pain[5] and there are a number of specific pain syndromes associated with breast cancer which require comprehensive assessment and management. Many patients survive for years with known skeletal metastases and the length of survival continues to increase for patients with metastatic disease. With the continuous advances in the management and treatment of these patients many are able to lead active and rewarding lives, living with a chronic illness.

The purpose of this chapter is to describe the main aspects of the assessment and management of pain and other complications from bone metastases such as, hypercalcaemia, pathological fractures, and spinal cord compression.

## Assessment and management of bone pain in advanced breast cancer

Multiple symptoms occur in advanced cancer and a simple assessment tool for each symptom is most appropriate for these patients. Assessment tools are useful to diagnose, to evaluate the intensity of the symptoms, to monitor the effectiveness of therapy, and to screen for side-effects of medications. Assessment tools should used regularly, especially when patients experience new symptoms, an increase in the intensity of pre-existing symptoms, or when therapy changes. The results should be documented in the patient's chart to ensure that symptoms are accurately monitored to facilitate effective treatment.

The therapeutic approach has to be multidimensional and individualized for each patient. Even patients with multiple and severe symptoms frequently have a good response to initial therapy. In these patients, a **unidimensional** approach (for example managing pain with opioids and nausea with antiemetics) can be appropriate. For those with persistent, severe symptoms, despite appropriate therapy (approximately 20% of patients with advanced cancer), a **multidimensional** evaluation should be performed.[6] Several assessment tools may be needed. Some examples are listed in (Table 9.1).[7–23]

### Pain assessment

The pain experience is multidimensional, with a complex interplay between pathophysiological, cognitive, and emotional influences.[24] Multidimensional assessment can be obtained with tools such as the Brief Pain Inventory (BPI)[10] or the Mc Gill Pain Questionnaire (MPQ),[11] and the Memorial Pain Assessment Card (MPAC).[9] Bone pain is the most commonly syndrome in patients with breast cancer and bone metastases (40–70%). The determination of the cause, type, and intensity of the pain

**Table 9.1** Multidimensional assessment

| Dimension | Tool |
| --- | --- |
| Symptom distress | Edmonton Symptom Assessment system (ESAS)[7] <br> Memorial Symptom Assessment Scale (MSAS)[8] |
| Pain | Memorial Pain Assessment Card (MPAC)[9] <br> Brief Pain Inventory (BPI)[10] <br> McGill Pain Questionnaire (MPQ)[11] |
| Delirium screening | Mini-Mental State Assessment (MMSE)[12,13] <br> Memorial Delirium Assessment Scale (MDAS)[14,15] <br> Confusion Assessment Method (CAM)[16,17] |
| Chemical coping | Attempts to Cut back on drink, being Annoyed at criticisms about drinking, feeling Guilty about drinking, and using alcohol as an Eye opener (CAGE)[18,19] <br> Michigan Alcoholism Screening Test (MAST)[20] |
| Physical function | Edmonton Functional Assessment Tool (EFAT)[21,22] <br> Functional Independence Measure (FIM)[23] |

are essential for the appropriate management of cancer pain. For those patients who have persistent pain in spite of appropriate therapy, multidimensional assessment is mandatory (Table 9.1).

There are three main pain syndromes that patients with breast cancer can experience: nociceptive, neuropathic, and incidental pain. The last two types of pain are usually more difficult to manage. The **nociceptive** pain mechanism occurs through the stimulation of nociceptors with afferent impulse propagated along the spinothalamic nociceptive pathways. Nociceptive pain is divided into somatic or visceral types. *Somatic* involves skin, bone, vessels, and mucosa. It is well localized and can be constant, waxing and waning, or intermittent. The pain quality can be gnawing, aching, and occasionally cramping. *Visceral* pain involves organs, is poorly localized and may possibly be referred. It is constant and is usually described by the patient as aching, squeezing, or cramping. Bone pain is most common somatic pain.

The mechanism of **neuropathic** pain is compression, invasion, destruction, or dysfunction of the CNS or peripheral nervous system. There are two types, dysaesthetic (e.g. deafferentation) and lancinating pain. *Dysaesthetic* pain is localized but may radiate (e.g. nerve root compression). It can be constant or waxing and waning, and may have a burning quality. *Lancinating* pain is paroxysmal, and the pain quality is sharp and shooting. Neuropathic pain is associated with spinal cord compression.

Finally, **incidental** pain is characterized by a severe increase in pain intensity with movements such as coughing, defecation, swallowing, or urination. It is commonly associated with malignant bone pain. Patients with neuropathic pain frequently require the administration of adjuvant drugs such as tricyclic antidepressants mainly used for dysaesthetic pain (nortriptyline, amitriptyline and others) or antiepileptics for the management of lancinating pain (gabapentin, lamotrigine and others).[25] The choice of anticonvulsant or antidepressant also depends on possible drug interactions with other medications in the patient's regimen, the effectiveness and tolerability of the drug for that individual, frequency of dosing, and patient preference. Transmucosal fentanyl may also be useful in the management of patients with incidental pain due to its rapid onset of action and short duration of effect.[26]

It will help the patient if the physician identifies early on the presence of pain characteristics that indicate that the pain will be difficult to manage. When there is a lack of awareness of these poor prognostic factors it can result in an unhelpful rapid escalation of medication, particularly of opioids, and subsequent toxicity problems (Table 9.2).[27]

## Pain treatment

The choice of which drug or drugs to use depends upon the severity of pain. Different types of pain tend to respond to different analgesics (Table 9.3).[28]

Opioids are the most effective treatment in patients with cancer pain[29] and because pain syndromes in cancer are unique in intensity and duration opioids are often required at the highest doses used in clinical medicine. There are several misconceptions about opioids that contribute to under-treatment of cancer pain;[30–32] these include unwarranted fears about addiction.

**Table 9.2** Poor prognosis factors for cancer pain control

| Factor | Worse prognosis | Better prognosis |
|---|---|---|
| Mechanism | Neuropathic | Nociceptive (somatic or visceral) |
| Nature | Incidental | Continuous |
| Psychological distress | Somatization (anxiety, depression) | Somatization absent |
| Opioid tolerance | >5% dose increase per day | <5% dose increase per day |
| History of alcoholism or drug abuse | Positive (CAGE ≥2, possibility of chemical coping) | Negative |

**Table 9.3** Treatment of cancer pain depends on the type and intensity

| Pain type | | Intensity | Treatment |
|---|---|---|---|
| Nociceptive | Bone, soft tissue | Mild, moderate Severe | Non-opioid (opioid if required) Opioid + non-opioid |
| | Visceral | Mild Moderate, severe | Non-opioid (opioid if required) Opioid + non-opioid |
| Neuropathic | Nerve compression Deafferentation | | Corticosteroid ± opioid Antidepressant or anticonvulsant |
| Incidental | | | Avoid pain-causing manoeuvres Rapid-acting opioids Bisphosphonates, orthopaedic procedures |

In cases of *mild pain*, physicians can start therapy with a non-opioid drug, such as acetaminophen, or with a weak opioid, such as codeine, or an NSAID. If the pain is not controlled with the starting dose, physicians should increase it. Weak opioids have a flat dose–response curve, because they have a therapeutic ceiling[33], contrary to strong opioids in which the analgesic effect increases as the dose increases so that toxicity becomes the only limiting factor in the dose escalation. Some preparations include combination of opioids with acetaminophen or NSAID. With these drugs the opioid dose escalation is limited by the toxicity of the associated drug. If there is no pain improvement as the dose is increased this indicates that a stronger (more potent) opioid is required.

*Moderate and severe pain* requires a stronger opioid at the outset, such as morphine, hydromorphone, oxycodone, methadone, or fentanyl.

### Opioid therapy initiation

Initiate pain therapy with a rapidly-acting/normal-release opioid (Table 9.4). The recommended starting dose should be titrated against pain severity, that is the dose should be increased as rapidly as needed over 3–4 days until the pain is controlled.

The increase of the daily opioid dose depends on the number of doses which are needed for breakthrough pain. If a patient needs more than three doses for break-

**Table 9.4** Rapid and long-acting strong opioids

| Opioid | Onset action | Half-life | Duration of action | Comments |
|---|---|---|---|---|
| **Agonist opioids, rapid-acting** | | | | |
| Morphine | 20–30 min | 1.5–4.5 h | 3–6 h | Metabolites (M6G) accumulation in renal failure; multiple routes of administration and formulations available |
| Hydromorphone | 20–30 min | 2–3 h | 4–5 h | Multiple routes of administration and formulations available |
| Diamorphine (heroin) | 10–30 min | 3 min | 3–4 h | Only available in the UK and Canada; more soluble than morphine and is favoured for subcutaneous route |
| Oxycodone | 20–30 min | 3.5–4.5 h | 4–6 h | Higher oral bioavailability than morphine (about 1.5–2 times) |
| Oral transmucosal fentanyl citrate | 3–5 min | 6–8 h | 2–3 h | Lollipops available to deliver 200, 400, 600, 800, 1200, 1600 μ/h |
| Pethidine (meperidine) | 20 min | 2–3 h | 5–6 h | Not recommended for routine use; contraindicated in patients with renal failure and receiving MAO inhibitors |
| **Agonist opioids, long-acting** | | | | |
| Fentanyl transdermal system | 3–23 h | 24 h | 48–72 h | Patches available to deliver 25,50,75,100 μg/h |
| Methadone | 30 min | 8–75 h | 4–24 h | The lipid-solubility and long half-life means that accumulation is bound to occur particularly in elderly patients |

through pain, the dose for the following day should be the sum of all the breakthrough pain doses plus the scheduled dose. There is no need to increase the daily scheduled dose when patients need fewer than three breakthrough pain doses.

In patients with severe pain, a higher starting dose may be needed. It is extremely important to avoid slow (modified) release preparation and opioids with a long half-life when starting opioid therapy. These opioids take time before they reach their full effect (up to 3 days in the case of methadone), and most patients need more rapid control of their pain. In addition, they are difficult to titrate and can accumulate, which causes toxicity, especially in patients with renal failure.

**Breakthrough pain:** Physicians should always prescribe rapidly-acting opioids for breakthrough pain (pain that is not controlled with the scheduled analgesics). The dose for breakthrough pain is usually 10% of the daily dose.[1]

**The adverse effects of opioids:** There are several troublesome side-effects of opioids. The most frequent are drowsiness, nausea, and constipation. The first two usually improve after 3 or 4 days of therapy but constipation does not. Therefore, it is a common practice to prescribe antiemetics, such as metoclopramide (for the first 3–4 days), and laxatives (as long as the opioid is used) to prevent and treat nausea and constipation respectively.

## Maintenance therapy

Once the pain is controlled, rapidly-acting (normal release) opioids can be switched to those of modified release preparations or to opioids with a longer half-life such as methadone. This is done primarily to give patients the convenience of taking fewer pills per day. They are not more effective and they do not have fewer side-effects. It is strongly recommended to switch to the modified release form of the same type of opioid (e.g. morphine to morphine-SR). If the physician switches to a different kind of opioid (e.g. morphine to hydromorphone-SR) the dose of the new opioid has to be reduced by approximately 30%.

**The fentanyl patch:** Special care must be taken when using the fentanyl patch as it takes many hours to reach its full effect. It is crucial to continue with the previously prescribed opioid (normal release) for approximately 12 h after a fentanyl patch is started and to monitor the patient carefully during this time for possible drowsiness and slow respiration or conversely for inadequate pain control. For the same reason, once the fentanyl patch is discontinued, physicians must wait about 12–18 h to start a new modified release or long-acting opioid with 'rescue' (normal release) preparation available to manage breakthrough pain. The calculated equianalgesic dose of fentanyl patch dose should not be reduced when switching from morphine because fentanyl's conversion table already takes into account incomplete cross-tolerance.

Sometimes, upward titration may be needed during opioid therapy because the disease has progressed. In other cases, when a patient with satisfactory pain control experiences opioid toxicity, or when the pain improves due to other treatments such

[1] Editor's note: in the UK it would normally be 1/6th of the total daily dose of morphine (or other opioid 4 hourly) but neither figure is an absolute and should be titrated for a given individual.

as radiotherapy, downward titration may be indicated. It is important to keep pain control under careful and regular review and give patients enough information to manage their pain effectively or seek help early if pain control is deteriorating.

## Opioid toxicity

The most common side-effects of opioids are sedation, nausea, and constipation. Sedation that persists after several days of opioid therapy and is severe can be treated with psychostimulants such as methylphenidate. The dose is 5–10 mg in the morning and 5 mg at noon.[34] Other less common side-effects include vertigo, pruritus, and urinary retention. There are some reports of pulmonary oedema in patients undergoing rapid titration for uncontrolled pain.[35] Opioids also produce neurotoxicity such as hallucinations, delirium, myoclonus (spasm of the extremities and facial muscles), and hyperalgesia.[36] Unfortunately, physicians are frequently unaware of these side-effects and they usually only make the diagnosis once patients exhibit gross symptoms. Patients on opioid therapy should be evaluated systematically for neurotoxicity.

Neurotoxicity is usually seen in patients taking a high dose of opioids, with prolonged administration, in those with previous borderline cognition, and in patients with renal failure.

**Renal insufficiency:** Special care has to be taken in patients with renal insufficiency because there is a high probability of metabolite accumulation in this condition. It is recommended that reduced doses of opioid are used and an 'as needed' regimen (at least initially), even in patients with no signs of opioid toxicity. The treatment of opioid-induced neurotoxicity consists of hydration (in an attempt to increase renal elimination of the parent drugs and its metabolites, appropriate to the patient's renal function or cardiac status), opioid rotation, that is changing the opioid used (see below), and, in some cases, opioid dose reduction. Physicians should also look for other causes of neurotoxicity and treat them accordingly.

## Opioid rotation

Opioid rotation is indicated when the pain is not under control despite high doses of an opioid, or when the patient's pain is adequately controlled but only on a large quantity of opioids (making administration difficult or impractical) or when tolerance or toxicity develops. When starting opioid rotation, consider the variations between individuals in opioid requirements, the lack of complete cross tolerance between opioids, and the fact that standard conversion tables were not developed for the purpose of opioid rotation.[37,38] Therefore, the calculated equianalgesic dose of the new opioid should be reduced by approximately 30–50% as a precaution and adequate doses of 'as needed' medication prescribed.

**Methadone:** Among opioids, methadone requires special consideration because of its unique characteristics.[39] It is considered a second-choice drug in the management of cancer pain and is widely used in the palliative care setting. Methadone is a synthetic, potent opioid agonist and acts through mu receptors. It also has an antagonist action on NMDA receptors, which play an important role in opioid tolerance, potentiation of opioid effects, and neuropathic pain. It has excellent bioavailability of approximately 80%. It is metabolized in the liver where it may interact with inducers and inhibitors of cytochrome P450 system. It has a long half-life, up to 190 h, and duration of action of 6–12 h, which allows physicians to administer it every 8–12 h. It is excreted by the faeces and has no active metabolites; therefore no adjustment is needed in patients with renal failure.

The onset of action is rapid but it takes time to reach its full effect, and so increasing the dose more frequently than every 3–4 days is not recommended. The conversion of methadone to other opioids is complex, and it varies with the dose of methadone in use at time of opioid switching. Physicians who are not familiar with methadone may inadvertently administer an overdose during opioid rotation and it should only be used with specialist advice. The overdose risk is increased in patients taking higher dose of their current opioid because conversion tables become more inaccurate (or approximate) at higher doses. The potency of methadone varies from 3 to 20 times that of morphine depending on the dose used. The higher the dose of morphine, the higher the potency methadone. Once patients have been successfully rotated to methadone, dose titration and monitoring are no different from those of other opioids.

Methadone is available in tablet, liquid, suppository and injectable forms. As it is 30–50 times cheaper than other opioids, physicians should consider methadone when cost is a concern. In many developing countries, opioid therapy is not adequately provided because it is relatively expensive and methadone may then play an important role.

**Table 9.5** Pain treatment according to mechanism

| Cause | | 1st line treatment | 2nd line treatment | To consider |
|---|---|---|---|---|
| Bone pain | | Primary analgesic: opioids, NSAIDs | Corticosteroids | Surgery (orthopaedic treatment) |
| | | | Bisphosphonates | Nerve block epidural |
| | | Palliative radiotherapy | Systemic radioisotopes | Transcutaneous electrical nerve stimulation (TENS) |
| Nerve pain | Compression | Primary analgesic: opioid | Radiotherapy | Nerve block |
| | | | Corticosteroids | Transcutaneous electrical nerve stimulation (TENS) |
| | | | Local anaesthetic | |
| | Deafferentation | Secondary analgesic: tricyclic antidepressant Anticonvulsant | Nerve block | |

**Table 9.6** Some adjuvant drugs in cancer pain

| Type | Examples | Indications | Dose |
|---|---|---|---|
| Antidepressant | Amitriptyline | Neuropathic pain | 10–25 mg P.O. titrated up to 150 mg |
| Anticonvulsant | Gabapentin | Neuropathic pain | 100 mg every 8 h up to 300 mg P.O. every 8 h (900 mg every 6 h may be required for severe cases) |
| Corticosteroids | Dexamethasone | Neuropathic pain, Bone and visceral pain | 10 mg po/sc/iv every 8 h and rapid decrease upon response |
| Bisphosphonates | Pamidronate Zoledronic acid | Bone pain and hypercalcaemia | 90 mg iv every 4 weeks 4–8 mg i.v. every 4 weeks |
| Anti-inflammatory | NSAIDs | Bone and inflammatory pain | Variable |

Opioids are the first line of therapy for advanced cancer patients. Sometimes the addition of adjuvant drugs can be useful to manage pain or opioid side-effects.[40,41] The use of adjuvant analgesics should be considered when it is not possible to achieve good analgesia and opioids have been titrated to the level of dose-limited toxicity (Table 9.5).

In addition to specific non-pharmacological therapies (such as TENS) and invasive analgesic techniques (such as nerve blockade), which may be useful, it is essential to remember that pain relief is more that using a series of techniques and requires multidimensional assessment and treatment including social, psychological, and spiritual care (see Chapter 2). We can summarize the breast cancer pain treatments according to the mechanism in Table 9.5.

## Specific pain syndromes in metastatic breast cancer

Most patients with advanced breast cancer have multiple causes and sites of pain. The most common cause of cancer pain (65–85%) is caused by direct involvement of the structures, by the primary or metastatic tumour.[42] In 15–25% of patients, the pain is related to anticancer therapy such as surgery, radiotherapy, and chemotherapy and 3–10% of the patients have pain unrelated to the cancer or its therapy (e.g. postherpetic neuralgia, arthritic pain, musculoskeletal).[28]

Breast cancer commonly metastasizes to bone and therefore patients have a high incidence of pain (70%).[43,44] Bone metastastes in breast cancer affect more than half of women during the course of their disease[45] and this also is the most common site of first distant relapse.[46,47] Patients thus affected have relatively long survival after the diagnosis of bone metastases compared with patients with extraosseous metastases. Their median survival is usually beyond 20 months, and about 10% of them are alive 5–10 years after the first diagnostic of bone metastases.[47] Bone metastases cause significant morbidity due to severe bone pain (70%), hypercalcaemia of malignancy (20–40%), pathological fractures (10–20%), and spinal cord or nerve root compression (5–10%).[48,49] The last two constitute a major cause of prolonged disability (45–75%) in breast cancer.[50,51]

## Bone metastases

Bone metastases develop by vascular spread starting in the vascular cavity of the bone and progressing by involving the cortex. Cancer cells cause bone destruction primarily by stimulation of osteoclast activity. Three principal disturbances of remodelling occur when bone has been infiltrated by a malignancy. First, increased bone turnover results in substantial deficits of cancellous bone (more than cortical bone). Second, an imbalance exists between the amounts of bone resorbed and formed. Third, a phenomenon called *uncoupling* occurs whereby erosion cavities are formed but are unable to repair themselves.[52]

Breast cancer bone metastases are predominantly osteolytic (50%) or mixed osteolytic and osteoblastic (40%), with only a small proportion (10%) being osteoblastic alone. Osteoclasts are primarily responsible for the bone resorption of lytic metastases, either through direct activation by tumour cells or via tumour-secreted factors such as cytokines and parathyroid hormone related peptide.[53]

Bone metastases occur predominantly (80%) in the axial skeleton, which contains the more vascular red marrow. Metastases occur most frequently in the vertebrae (especially thoracic spine), ribs, pelvis, and femur. The main complication of vertebral metastases is vertebrae collapse, radiculopathy, and epidural spinal cord compression.[47–49]

Malignant bone pain syndrome consists of a triad of background pain, spontaneous pain, and movement-induced or incidental pain.[54,55] The *background or continuous pain* is the most frequent presentation of bone pain, and it may be well localized to one or more specific bone areas or is poorly localized. It usually develops gradually over a period of weeks or months, becoming progressively severe in intensity. This pain has been described as dull or as a deep boring sensation that aches or burns, often accompanied by episodes of stabbing discomfort. The *spontaneous* pain consists of intermittent episodes of intense pain without apparent triggering events. The *movement-induced or incidental pain* consists of intermittent episodes of intense pain upon movement – standing and walking often aggravate pain. These episodes often occur with increased pressure on the area, which may account for its worsening by night and the fact that it may not necessarily be relieved by lying down or by sleep.[56,61]

Diagnosis of bone pain can usually be made by history and physical examination. The physicians should enquire about the onset, quality, intensity, localization, radiation of the pain, factors that exacerbate or alleviate the pain, and other systematic symptoms such as bowel and urinary problems and functional problems. A musculoskeletal and neurological examination must be completed, focussing on palpable tenderness in the skeletal system and neurological deficits and alterations. Back pain without weakness of the limbs, paraesthesiase, sensory change, or bladder or bowel impairment should be carefully assessed for potential spinal cord compression. It is important to note that the differential diagnosis of bone pain includes degenerative disease due to osteoporosis in elderly women with acute back due to collapsed vertebrae.

**Table 9.7** Imaging tests for detecting bone metastases[57–60]

| Test | Advantages | Disadvantages |
|------|-----------|---------------|
| X-ray (plain radiography) | Confirm symptomatic lesions (trabecular and cortical bone) | Delayed appearance: metastases lesions may not appear for several months (30–75% bone must be lost before lesions become apparent)[57] |
| | Less expensive Assessment of risk for pathological fracture | |
| Bone scan (scintigraphy) | Screening tool (rapid whole-body images at a reasonable cost)[58] | Low specificity (positive in osteoarthritis, infections, trauma, and Paget) Negative in purely lytic lesions |
| | Detects new lesions | |
| CT (computed tomography) | Evaluates cortical, trabecular, and marrowbone Detect metastases in the marrow before bone destruction becomes evident[59] | Relatively expensive |
| MRI (magnetic resonance imaging) | Better contrast resolution than CT for visualizing soft tissue and spinal cord compression[60] | Expensive |
| PET scan (positron emission tomography) | Detects early new marrow lesions of soft tissue and bone metastases | Very expensive Lack of availability Limited use in palliative care setting[58] |

**Table 9.8** Therapies for management of malignant bone pain

| Therapy | Onset | Effect |
|---------|-------|--------|
| **Systemic** | | |
| Opioids | Immediate | Analgesia |
| NSAIDs | Immediate to days | Analgesia + anti-inflammatories |
| Corticosteroids | Immediate to days | Analgesia + anti-inflammatories |
| Bisphosphonates | Days to weeks | Suppression of osteoclasts + some analgesia |
| Hormone and chemotherapy | Days to weeks | Tumour shrinkage + analgesia |
| Radiopharmaceuticals | Weeks | Tumour shrinkage + analgesia |
| **Local** | | |
| Radiotherapy | Weeks | Tumour shrinkage + analgesia |
| Surgery | Immediate to days | Prevent further fracture |

The imaging tests (X-ray, bone scan, CT, MRI, and PET) should be interpreted in conjunction with the clinical picture (Table 9.7).[57–60]

The goals of treatment for bone metastases are:

◆ to control pain;
◆ restore mobility;
◆ prevent pathological fractures;
◆ prevent neurological complications;
◆ prevent, or intervene early in, hypercalcaemia or myelosuppression.

Palliative interventions include analgesia, hormone therapy, chemotherapy, surgery, radiation therapy, including radiopharmaceuticals, and bisphosphonate therapy.

1 **Analgesics** – in moderate to severe pain opioids are a good option for control of diffuse pain and pain in isolated areas of bone, and may commonly involve combination treatment regimens, including the use of other relatively low cost drugs such as corticosteroids and NSAIDs. Other, higher-cost therapies are explained below (Table 9.8).

2 **Hormone and chemotherapy hormone blockade** is used with the intention of depriving hormonally dependent tumours of their stimulus, thus slowing tumour growth.[62] Oestrogen blockers, such as tamoxifen, are commonly used. Assessing the independent impact of chemotherapy on quality of life and actual pain relief of bone metastases is difficult because other treatments are generally administered at the same time.[63] Unfortunately, less than 50% of patients benefit from currently available endocrine or cytotoxic chemotherapy.[64,65]

3 **Radiotherapy** is clearly effective at reducing pain from painful bone metastases. External beam radiation directly kills tumour cells and also may have an effect on the chemical mediators of pain (such as substance P) at the bone site.[62] This is the first treatment used for a solitary bone metastasis.[66] For most patients, a single dose or a short course of 1 to 2 weeks is sufficient to give pain relief with minimal side-effects. Multiple lesions may be treated with wide-field irradiation (e.g. hemibody radiation, treating the upper or lower half of the body), although an increased incidence of side-effects exists with this method. The overall pain response rates for single fraction and multifraction radiotherapy is about 60%; there is no evidence of any difference in efficacy between different fraction schedules. However, the retreatment rate and pathological fracture rates are higher after single-fraction radiotherapy.[67] Single-fraction radiotherapy may have a significant role in the palliative setting.[68] Studies with quality-of-life and health economic end points are warranted to find out the optimal treatment options for each clinical situation. Prophylactic radiation may be used to prevent an impending fracture, with or without surgery.

4 **Radiopharmaceuticals** are bone seeking (site-selective radioisotopes). They can offer pain relief for multiple sites of malignant bone lesions. They are convenient and generally less toxic than external beam radiation. Strontium 89 is chemically similar to calcium, has a preferential affinity for osteoblastic lesions, and delivers therapeutic amounts of beta radiation. Samarium 153, once taken up

**Table 9.9** Bisphosphonates approved for treatment of patients with bone metastases from breast cancer[113–115]

| Type | Relative potency | Via/schedule | Time of infusion (iv) | Results |
|---|---|---|---|---|
| **First generation: non-nitrogen** | | | | |
| Clodronate[a] | 1 | Oral/ daily sc/ iv every 3–4 weeks | 2–3 h | Increased time to first SRE Improved quality of life[73] |
| **Second generation: single nitrogen** | | | | |
| Pamidronate[b] | 20 | iv | 2–4 h | Reduced proportion experiencing SRE; Delay in first SRE[74] |
| | | every 3–4 weeks | | |
| Ibandronate[a] | 857 | Oral/ daily iv every 3–4 weeks | 1 h | Reduced SMR[75] |
| **Third generation: two nitrogens** | | | | |
| Zoledronic[b] acid | 16 700 | iv every 3–4 weeks | 15 min | 20% risk reduction for a SRE[76] |

SRE, skeletal-related event; SMR, skeletal mobility rates; iv, intravenous; sc, subcutaneous.
[a]Approved in Europe.

by the target bone lesions, emits beta and gamma radiation. Less exposure of healthy tissue occurs with samarium than with strontium because it is less penetrating, making it the radiopharmaceutical of choice.[69] In a recent retrospective study of Sapienza and colleagues, which evaluated the bone pain palliation after samarium 153 therapy, the reduction obtained in pain scores with samarium (75% to 100%) ws the 49% [65] and mild-moderate myelosuppresion was present in 75.3% of the patients, but was usually recovered at 8 weeks [65]. In a 2003 Cochrane review of four randomized and controlled trials of 325 patients with metastatic bone pain that compared treatment with radioisotopes and placebo, indicated that there is some evidence that radioisotopes may give complete reduction in pain over one to six months with no increase in analgesic use, but adverse effects, specifically leukocytopenia and thrombocytopenia, have also been experienced[66].

5 **Bisphosphonates** (Table 9.9) are an important alternative for bone pain where radiation tolerance has been reached or radiotherapy is not readily available.[66] The role of the bisphosphonates in breast cancer has been reviewed recently because these agents have an increasing role in oncology, not only in the management of metastatic bone disease (as an effective supplementary approach to radiotherapy) and skeletal complications,[72] but also for prevention of cancer-treatment-induced bone loss (frequent in long survivors, secondary to treatments).[73] Bisphosphonates inhibit osteoclastic resorption[74] and they have become standard treatment for tumour-induced hypercalcaemia.[75] Recent, controlled trials have shown that bisphosphonates reduce bone pain,[76] improve quality of life,[77] and reduce the

number of and time of skeletal events.[78–81] A current Cochrane Review of bisphosphonates in women with early and advanced breast cancer concludes that in advanced breast cancer and clinically evident bone metastases, the use of bisphosphonates (oral or intravenous) in addition to hormone therapy or chemotherapy, when compared with placebo or no bisphosphonates, reduces the risk of developing skeletal events and increases the time to a skeletal event. Bisphosphonates may also reduce bone pain in women with advanced breast cancer and clinically evident bone metastases. In women with early breast cancer, the effectiveness of oral clodronate in reducing the evidence of bone metastases remains an open question needing further research.[76] Another systematic review supports the efficacy of bisphosphonates in providing some pain relief for bone metastases but also concludes that there is insufficient evidence to recommend it for immediate pain relief or as first-line therapy.[77] This topic is discussed in detail in Chapter 8.

6 **Surgical management** is extremely effective in alleviating pain.[46] Vertebroplasty and kyphoplasty are minimal invasive procedures used for vertebral compression fractures. They both attempt to stabilize trabecular microfractures via cement interdigitation. Vertebroplasty was first used to treat osteoporotic compression fractures in 1995.[82] This procedure involves using a large-bore needle to cannulate the pedicle, followed by injection of polymethylmethacrylate into the vertebral body. Many investigators have reported successful outcomes with this technique with regard to immediate pain relief,[83] although there was a high incidence of complications, especially epidural leakage of cement outside of vertebral bodies. Kyphoplasty is a relative new procedure evolving from vertebroplasty and its clinical efficacy was first described in 2001. This technique combines injection of polymethilmethacrylate to strengthen a vertebra with balloon angioplasty, and has minimum complication because a specific void is created, the injection pressure is lower, and the bone-filler viscosity can be higher, which reduces the incidence of cement leakage.[84]

7 **Percutaneous image-guided radiofrequency ablation** (RFA) of pathologic fractures (ablation that uses heat energy to destroy the tumour) is now being studied in metastatic bone lesions. It is a localized treatment that does not require general anaesthesia.[85] A small study in patients with painful osteolytic metastases suggests that this therapy may have a role in reducing malignant bone pain, reducing opioid requirement, and preventing the painful consequence of disease progression.[86]

8 **Invasive pain therapy** techniques should be considered, in a small minority of patients, when local and/or systemic therapy and adequate use of analgesics fails to provide adequate pain relief in malignant bone pain (see Chapter 2).

Patients with bone metastases can survive for years after diagnosis. Rehabilitation strategies should incorporate safety as well as strengthening and mobility measures. The use of orthotics, such as walkers, braces, and collars, exercises that focus on bone protection and increasing muscle strength, and home environment modifications can assist in reaching these goals.[87]

## Hypercalcaemia

Hypercalcaemia occurs in 20–40% of patients with breast cancer,[88] which is more frequent than in general malignant disease (10–20%).[89]

Metastases within the bone itself may have a local effect on bone resorption, and also the solid tumours secrete calcaemic factors that act both on the skeleton to increase bone resorption, and on the kidney to increase conservation of calcium. There is no correlation between the presence and degree of bony metastases and incidence of hypercalcaemia.[90] The picture may be mixed, but the majority (90%) of patients with solid tumours will have evidence of a humoral component contributing to the elevation, irrespective of whether bone metastases are present or not.[91]

Clinical manifestations of hypercalcaemia are varied and are often related to the rapidity of onset of hypercalcaemia, and therefore someone with mildly elevated calcium can be symptomatic whilst another with moderately elevated calcium is asymptomatic. Symptoms can be divided into gastrointestinal (anorexia, nausea and vomiting, and constipation), renal (polyuria and polydipsia and rarely nephorocalcinosis), and neurological effects (confusion, drowsiness, and coma).[92]

There are four aims of treatment:

1  correction of dehydration;
2  inhibition of bone resorption;
3  increasing renal excretion of calcium;
4  the treatment of the underlying malignancy.

Rehydration itself may correct mild hypercalcaemia simply by increasing the intravascular volume and promoting hypercalciuria.[93] Treatment of the underlying malignancy is the single most important factor in determining prognosis in the patients.[94] There are a number of different drugs that have been used in the treatment of hypercalcaemia apart from bisphosphonates but the latter are now the drugs of choice. Bisphosphonates normalize serum calcium in >70% of patients with hypercalcaemia of malignancy within 2–6 days.[95]

## Pathological fractures

The axial skeleton is commonest site for bony metastases although the great majority of those in which surgical intervention are carried out involve the appendicular skeleton (femur, humerus, and acetabulum). There is a trend in modern surgical practice, however, towards increasing intervention for spinal metastases.

The role of the orthopaedic surgeon in the management of bone metastases falls into three principles categories:

1  prophylactic fixation of metastatic deposits where there is a risk of fracture;
2  stabilization or reconstruction following pathological fracture;
3  decompression of spinal cord and nerve roots, followed by stabilization of the affected vertebrae.

### Appendicular skeleton

For some patients, the first presentation of bone metastases will be with a pathological fracture of the appendicular skeleton (in response to a low energy injury); the most common site of symptomatic fracture is the proximal femur.

Radiographs should be taken of any lesion in weight-bearing bones, to aid assessment of the risk of pathological fracture. As an increasing amount of bone cortex is lost the risk of fracture rises steeply and, once 50% of the bone cortex is lost in any radiological projection, fracture should be regarded as inevitable,[96,97] and prophylactic fixation should be performed prior to the administration of radiotherapy.[98] Postoperative therapy has been associated with a decrease in the need for second surgical procedures and improved functional status of patients with previously unirradiated long bone and acetabular lesions.[99] Treatment is started within 2 to 4 weeks of surgery.

Where there is less than 50% cortical erosion, radiotherapy may be considered without prophylactic fixation, the exception being the femoral neck where any degree of cortical erosion should be considered as an indication for prophylactic fixation. Non-weight-bearing bones, such as the ribs, fibula, and much of the pelvis, can safety be treated with radiotherapy alone in most cases.[99]

### Axial skeleton

In spinal metastatic disease, those who are most likely to benefit from surgery, and thus in most need of a specialist orthopaedic opinion, are those who have one or more of the following features:

- pain exacerbated by movement and relieved on rest (spinal instability);
- 50% of vertebral or vertebral body destruction;
- moderate deformity and collapse.[98]

Certain sites are at particular risk of fracture in the presence of bone metastases and disease progression. For example there is a 28% risk of pathological fracture occurring through a given cervical spine metastasis in a 4-week period in which there is no response to either systemic or local treatment.[99]

The presence of significant soft-tissue metastases (liver, lung, brain, etc.) may affect management decisions. Where the life expectancy is assumed to be less than 6 weeks, the multidisciplinary team should give careful consideration before embarking on any major surgical procedure. The patient's wishes are, of course, central to any decision. Against that, it must be borne in mind that a patient immobilized by bone metastases will have an extremely poor quality of life, and will not improve or regain mobility without surgery.[100,101] Spinal cord compression is an emergency and is discussed separately below.

## Spinal cord compression

Spinal cord compression (SCC) from epidural metastases occurs in 5–10% of cancer patients within the last 2 years of illness[102] and up to 40% of patients with pre-existing non-spinal bone metastases.[103] Of those with bony spinal disease, 10–20% develop symptomatic spinal cord compression, resulting in over 25 000 cases per year, and number is expected to grow.[104]

The thoracic spine is the most common site of disease (70%), followed by the lumbar spine (20%), and cervical spine (10%).[104] Metastatic spine disease can arise from one of three locations: the vertebral column (85%), the paravertebral region

(10–15%), and, rarely, the epidural or subarachnoid/ intramedullary space itself (<5%).[104] Multiple lesions at non-contiguous levels occur in 10–40% of cases.[103–105]

The clinical presentation of SCC depends on the severity: an acute onset is likely to involve severe pain with motor and sensory deficits and bowel and bladder dysfunction. Pain at the time of the diagnosis for a median of 8 weeks is reported by 83–95% of patients. It may be worse after a period of lying down because of distension of the epidural plexus, and may be more persistent with intradural lesions. Over time, pain may become more radicular, especially with involvement of lumbosacral spine. Weakness at the time of diagnosis is present in 60–85% of patients, and sensory deficits are slightly less common than weakness (40–90%) and patients tend to be less aware. Bowel and bladder dysfunction tend to occur late and it is important to make the diagnosis, where possible, before this has occurred.[106]

Clinically suspected SCC must be confirmed by imaging, not only to define the diagnosis but also to make informed decisions about treatment. SCC is an oncological emergency and early recognition and treatment of spinal cord compression will preserve ambulation and continence. If the patient is treated while he or she is still ambulant, the probability of retaining the ability to walk is 89–94%.[107] If the patient becomes paraparetic before treatment, the probability of being able to walk again is only 39–51%, and if he or she becomes paralyzed, it decreases to 10%.[106] Emergency magnetic resonance imaging of the entire spine is needed (or CT myelogram if MRI is contraindicated, but this is associated with more complications and is not as sensitive).[107,108]

The type of treatment chosen will depend on many factors, including the site and number of levels, whether the compression is partial or complete, fixability, duration, performance status, and predicted survival. Treatment options are steroids plus radiotherapy (for most patients) or steroids plus surgery and radiotherapy (for selected patients):

1 **Corticosteroid therapy** decreases cord oedema[106,109] and pain, helps preserve neurological function, and improves overall outcome after specific therapy.[110] Steroids are usually recommended for a short period, to be reassessed and stopped or tailed off as appropriate after surgical decompression or the completion of radiotherapy. Steroid treatment must be accompanied by gastro-protection. High-dose dexamethasone (100 mg iv bolus followed by 24 mg orally four times daily for 3 days, then tapered over 10 days)[2] is probably indicated for patients with impaired function of the spinal cord or cauda equina or with high-grade radiological lesion. At this dose, the drug substantially increases the number of these patients who remain ambulatory (81% compared with 63%).[110] Other patients usually receive lower-dose regimens (10 mg iv followed by 4 mg iv four times daily, then tapered over 14 days), which are better tolerated[107] but many not improve the chance of remaining ambulatory (57.1% compared with 57.9%).[111]

2 **Radiation in conjunction with high-dose steroids** is the non-invasive treatment of choice for spinal cord compressions because of its rapid results.[112] Radiotherapy is effective in the prevention of further tumour growth and neurological damage in most patients; it also ameliorates the pain.[107] About 70–80% of spine metastases

[2] It is important to follow local guidelines if considering high-dose steroids.

from breast cancer respond to radiotherapy.[112,113] Various dose schedules have been tried for pain relief and the reversal of compression. The most commonly used prescriptions are 30 Gy in 10 fractions and 8 Gy as a single fraction. Postoperative radiotherapy is generally recommended after decompression of the spinal cord or stabilization of the spine. In cervical thoracic spine a direct posterior field is used, giving 20 Gy in five fractions. In lumbar spine usually a single posterior field is employed. Radiotherapy is an excellent adjuvant to surgery and may be used as the only management in patients who are unsuitable for surgery or when palliation is the aim.

3 **Surgery decompression** is indicated with a mechanical stabilisation of the vertebral column to treat a single site of suspected involvement,[107] to treat progression despite radiation therapy,[114] or to treat vertebral instability, collapse with bone impinging on the spinal cord, or displacement.[107] Ambulatory patients are equally likely to remain ambulatory with radiation therapy or laminectomy.[113–115] In the case of rapid-onset SCC, when surgery is indicated, the aim should be to commence surgery within 12 hours (speed of onset bears an important relation to response). Neurological recovery is dependent on the rapidity of neurological decline, duration of neurological decline, and, most importantly, neurological status before treatment. Recently, minimally invasive surgical techniques, such as kyphoplasty/ vertebroplasty and stereotactic radiosurgery have been added to the surgeon's armamentarium. In a recent randomized controlled trial comparing direct decompressive surgical resection followed by adjuvant radiation with conventional radiation alone (both groups were treated with the same steroid protocol and both received the same total dose radiation dose), patients treated with minimal invasive surgery retained ambulatory and sphincter function significantly longer than patients in the radiation group.[116] Also, 56% of immobile patients in the surgical group regained the ability to walk compared with 19% in the radiation group. This study shows, for the first time, an undisputed advantage for surgery, where the goal is to achieve complete spinal cord decompression, over radiation therapy, which has been treatment of choice for the last 25 years. However, there are substantial potential complications, which must be considered (wound infections, cerebrospinal fluid fistulae, pneumonia, etc.).[117] Management decisions should be based on the patient's choice, clinical assessment and good quality imaging.

## Management of spinal cord compression

The importance of early diagnosis and prompt, effective treatment cannot be over-stated in this condition.[121,122] Although it was once thought that patients with SCC and paraplegia survived a median of 2–4 months after diagnosis it is now apparent that a significant proportion[121] live for a year or more with difficult symptoms and completely dependent on care; they are invisible to most oncology follow-up as practical difficulties preclude attendance at outpatient clinics. All oncology centres need to have policies and procedures in place to help early diagnosis and treatment in their area.

## Key points

◆ With improvements in treatment, many patients live longer with breast cancer and develop bony metastases.

◆ Bony metastases are a cause of significant morbidity in women with breast cancer, having a deleterious impact on quality of life.

◆ The most important complications are pain, hypercalcaemia, and spinal cord compression.

◆ A systematic approach must be used in the treatment of bone pain with regular review of therapy and goals of care.

◆ It is essential to diagnose spinal cord compression before neurological impairment to prevent catastrophic complications such as paraplegia.

◆ Bisphosphonates have had an important impact on improving quality of life for patients with bony metastases and breast cancer.

## References

1 Key, T.J., Verkasalo, P.K., and Banks, E. (2001). Epidemiology of breast cancer. *Lancet Oncol*, 2, 133–140.

2 American Cancer Society (1999). *Cancer facts and figures*. Atlanta, GA, American Cancer Society.

3 Parkin, D. M., Bray, F., Ferlay Metal (2005). Global cancer statistics, 2002. *CA Cancer J Clin*, 55, 74–108.

4 Falk, R.T., Fears, T.R., and Hoover, R.N. (2002). Does place of birth influence endogenous hormone levels in Asian-American women? *Br J Cancer*, 87, 54–60.

5 Vaino, A. and Auvinen, A. (1996). Prevalence of symptoms among patients with advanced cancer: an international collaborative study. *J Pain Symptom Manage*, 12, 3–10.

6 Kim, H.N., Bruera, E., and Jenkins, R. (2004). Symptom control and palliative care. In Cavalli, F., Hansen, H., and Kayne, S.B., eds. *Textbook of medical oncology*, 3rd edn, pp. 353–370. Taylor and Francis, New York.

7 Bruera, E., Kuehn, N., Miller, M.J., Selmser, P., and Macmillan, K. (1991). The Edmonton Symptom Assessment System (ESAS): a simple method for the assessment of palliative care patients. *J Palliat Care*, 7, 6–9.

8 Portenoy, R.K., Thaler, H.T., and Kornblith, A.B. (1994). The memorial symptom assessment scale: an instrument for the evaluation of symptom prevalence, characteristics and distress. *Eur J Cancer*, 30A, 1326–1336.

9 Fishman, B., Pasternak, S., and Wallenstein, S.L. (1983). The Memorial Pain Assessment Card: A valid instrument for the evaluation of cancer pain. *Cancer*, 60, 1151–1158.

10 Dault, R.L., Cleeland, C.S., and Flanery, R.C. (1983). Development of the Wisconsin Brief Pain Questionnaire to assess pain in cancer and other diseases. *Pain*, 17, 197–210.

11 Melazack, R. (1975). The McGill Pain Questionnaire: Major properties and scoring methods. *Pain*, 1, 277–299.

12 Folstein, M.F., Folstein, S.E., and McHugh, P.R. (1975). "Mini-mental state". A practical method for grading the cognitive state of patients for the clinician. *J Psychiatr Res*, 12, 189–198.

13 Lawlor, P.G. (2000). Occurrence, causes, and outcome of delirium in patients with advanced cancer: a prospective study. *Arch Intern Med*, 160, 786–794.

14 Lawlor, P.G., Nekolaichuck, C., Gagnon, B., Mancini, I.L., Pereira, J.L., and Bruera, E. (2000). Clinical Utility, Factor Analysis, and Further Validation of the Memorial Delirium Assessment Scale in Patients With advanced Cancer. *Cancer*, **88**, 2859–67.

15 Breitbart, W., Barry, R., Roth, A., Smith, M.J., Cohen, K., and Passik, S. (1997). The Memorial Assessment Scale. *J Pain Symptom Manage*, **13**, 128–137.

16 Laurila, J.V., Pitkala, K.H., Strandberg, T.E., and Tilvis, R.S. (2002). Confusion assessment method in the diagnostic of delirium among aged hospital patients: would it serve better in screening than as a diagnostic instrument? *Int J Geriatr Psychiatry*, **17**, 1112–1119.

17 Inouye, S.K., Van Dick, C.H., Alessi, C.A., Balkin, S., Siegal, A.P., and Horwitz, R.I. (1990). Clarifying confusion: the confusion assessment method. A new method for detection of delirium. *Ann Intern Med*, **113**, 941–948.

18 Moore, R., *et al.* (1989). Prevention, detection, and treatment of alcoholism in hospitalized patients. *JAMA*, **261**, 403–407.

19 Bruera, E., Moyano, J., Seifert, L., Fainsinger, R.L., Hanson, J., and Suarez-Almazor, M. (1995). The frequency of alcoholism among patients with pain due to terminal cancer. *J Pain Symptom Manage*, **10**, 599–603.

20 Gibbs, L.E. (1983). Validity and revalidate of the Michigan alcoholism screening test, a review. *Drug Alcohol Depend*, **12**, 279–285.

21 Kaasa, T. and Wessel, J. (1997). The Edmonton Functional Assessment Tool: preliminary development and evaluation for use in palliative care. *J Pain Symptom Manage*, **13**, 10–19.

22 Kaasa, T. and Wessel, J. (2001). The Edmonton Functional Assessment Tool: further development and validation for use in palliative care. *J Palliat Care*, **17**, 5–11.

23 Keith, R.A., Granger, C.V., Hamilton, B.B., and Sherwin, F.S. (1987). The functional independence measure: a new tool for rehabilitation. *Adv Clin Rehabil*, **1**, 6–18.

24 Ahles, T.A., Blanchard, E.B., and Ruckdeschel, J.C. (1993). The multidimensional nature of cancer-related pain. *Pain*, **17**, 277–288.

25 Bruera, E. and Ripamonti, E. (1993). Adjuvants to opioids analgesics. In Patt, R. ed., *Cancer pain*, pp. 142. Philadelphia, JB Lippincott.

26 Coluzzi, P.H. (2001). Breakthrough cancer pain: a randomized trial comparing oral trans-mucosal fentanyl citrate (OTFC) and morphine sulfate immediate release (MSIR). *Pain*, **91**, 123–130.

27 Hwang, S.S., *et al.* (2002). Development of a cancer pain prognostic scale. *J Pain Symptom Manage*, **24**, 366–378.

28 Cleary, J.F. (2000). Cancer Pain Management. *Cancer Control*, **7**, 120–131.

29 Foley, K. (1985). The treatment of cancer pain. *N Engl J Med*, **313**, 84–95.

30 Portenoy, R. and Payne, R. (1997). Acute chronic pain management. In Lowinson, J., Ruiz, P., and Millman, R., eds. *Comprehensive textbook of substance abuse*, p. 568. Baltimore, Williams and Wilkins.

31 Savage, S.R. (2003). Definitions related to the medical use of opioids: Evolution towards universal agreement. *J Pain Symptom Manage*, **26**, 655–667.

32 Payne, R. (2002). Opioid pharmacotherapy. In Berger, A., Portenoy, R., and Weissman, D. eds. *Principle and practice of palliative care and supportive oncology*, p. 289. Philadelphia, Lippincott William and Wilkins.

33 Twycross R., Wilcock A., Thorp S., Analgesics: Weak Opioids. In: Palliative Care Formulary PCF1. Oxon. England: Radcliffe Medical Press 1999, **5**: 100–101.

34  Bruera, E., Fainsinger, R., MacEachern, T., and Hanson, J. (1992). The use of methylphe-
    nidate in patients with incident cancer pain receiving regular opiates. A preliminary report.
    *Pain*, 50, 75–77.

35  Bruera, E. and Miller, M.J. (1989). Non-cardiogenic pulmonary edema after narcotic
    treatment for cancer pain. *Pain*, 39, 297–300.

36  Ripamonti, C. and Bruera, E. (1997). CNS Adverse effects of opioids in cancer patients.
    Guidelines for treatment. *CNS Drugs*, 8, 21–37.

37  Ripamonti, C., De Conno, F., Groff, L., Belzile, M., Pereira, J., Hanson, J., and Bruera, E.
    (1998). Equianalgesic dose/ratio between methadone and other opioid agonists in cancer
    pain: comparison of two clinical experiences. *Ann Oncol*, 9, 79–83.

38  Lawlor, P., Turner, K., Hanson, J., and Bruera, E. (1997). Dose ratio between morphine and
    hydromorphone in patients with cancer pain: a retrospective study. *Pain*, 72, 79–85.

39  Ayonrinde, O.T. and Bridge D.T. (2000). The rediscovery of methadone for cancer pain
    management. *Med J Aust*, 173, 536–540.

40  Mercadante, S. and Portenoy, R.K. (2001). Opioid poorly-responsive cancer pain. Part 1:
    clinical considerations. *J Pain Symptom Manage*, 21, 144–150.

41  Mercadante, S. and Portenoy, R.K. (2001). Opioid poorly-responsive cancer pain. Part 2:
    basic mechanisms that could shift dose response for analgesia. *J Pain Symptom Manage*, 21,
    255–264.

42  Foley, K. (1979). Pain syndrome in patients with cancer. In Bonica, J. and Ventafridda, V.,
    eds. *Advances in pain research and therapy*, p. 59. New York, Raven Press.

43  Nielsen, O.S., Munro, A.J., and Tannock, I.F. (1991). Bone metastases: pathophysiology and
    management policy. *J Clin Oncol*, 9, 509–524.

44  Pereira, J.;(1998). Management of bone pain. In Portenoy, R. and Bruera, E., eds. *Topics in
    palliative care*, vol 3, pp. 79–116. New York, Oxford University Press.

45  Scheid, V., Budar, A.U., Smith, T.L., and Hortobagyi, G.N. (1986). Clinical course of breast
    cancer patients with osseous metastases treated with combination chemotherapy. *Cancer*,
    58, 2589–2593.

46  Coleman, R.E. and Rubens, R.D. (1987). The clinical course of the bone metastases from
    breast cancer. *Br J Cancer*, 55, 61–66.

47  Galasko, C.S.B. (1986). Skeletal metastases. *Clin Orthop*, 210, 18–30.

48  Cowap, J., Hardy, J.R., and Roger, A. (2000). Outcome of malignant spinal cord compres-
    sion at a cancer center: implications for palliative care cervices. *J Pain Symptom Manage*, 19,
    257–264.

49  Helweg-Larsen, S. and Srensen, P.S. (1994). Symptoms and signs in metastatic spinal cord
    compression: A study of progression from first symptom until diagnosis in 153 patients. *Eur
    J Cancer*, 30A, 396–398.

50  Fidler, M.W. (1981). Incidence of fracture through metastases in long bones. *Acta Orthop
    Scand*, 52, 623–627.

51  Body, J., Lossignol, D., and Ronsen, A. (1997). The concept of rehabilitation of cancer
    patients. *Curr Opin Oncol*, 9, 332–340.

52  Kanis, J.A. and McCloskey, E.V. (1997). Bone turnover and biochemical markers in malig-
    nancy. *Cancer*, 80 (Suppl.), 1538–1545.

53  Coleman, R.E. and Rubens, R.D. (1985). Bone metastases and breast cancer. *Cancer Treat
    Reviews*, 12, 251–270.

54  Porteroy, R.K., Payne, D., and Jacobson, P. (1999). Breakthrough pain: characteristics and impact in patients with cancer pain. *Pain*, 81,129–134.

55  Meracdante, S. and Arcuri, E. (1998). Breakthrough pain in cancer patients: pathophysiology and treatment. *Cancer Treat Rev*, 24, 425–432.

56  Mundy, G.R. (1997). Mechanisms of bone metastases. *Cancer*, 80, 1546–1556.

57  Vinholes J., Coleman R., Eastell R.(1996) Effects of bone metastases on bone metabolism: implications for diagnosis, imaging and assessment of response to cancer treatment. *Cancer Treat Res*, 22, 289–331.

58  Hamaoka T., Madewell J.E., Podoloff D.A., Hortobagyi G.N. (2004) Bone imaging in metastatic breast cancer. *Journal of clinical Oncology*, 22, 2942–53.

59  Ryback L.D., Rosenthal D.I.(2001)Radiological imaging for the diagnosis of bone metastases.Q *J Nucl Med*, 45, 53–64.

60  Tryciecky E.W., Cottschalk A., Ludema K.(1997) Oncologic imaging: interactions of nuclear medicine with CT and MRI using the bone scan as a model. Semin Nucl Med, 27,142–51.

61  Portenoy, R.K. and Hagen, N.A. (1990). Breakthrough pain: Definition, prevalence and characteristics. *Pain*, 41, 273–281.

62  Mercadante, S. (1997). Malignant bone pain: Pathophysiology and treatment. *Pain*, 69, 1–18.

63  Nielsen, O.S., Munro, A.J., and Tannock, I.F. (1991). Bone metastases: Pathophysiology and management policy. *J Clin Oncol*, 9, 509–524.

64  Houston, S.J. and Rubens, R.D. (1995). The systemic treatment of bone metastases. *Clin Orthop*, 312, 95–104.

65  Janjan, N. (2001). Bone metastases: approaches to management. *Semin Oncol*, 28 (Suppl.), 28–34.

66  Hoskin, P.J. (2003). Bisphosphonates and radiation therapy for palliation of metastatic bone disease. *Cancer Treat Rev*, 29, 321–327.

67  Wai, M.S., Mike, S., Ines, H., and Malcolm, M. (2004). Palliation of metastatic bone pain: single fraction versus multifraction radiotherapy- a systematic review of the randomized trials. *Cochrane Database Syst Rev*, 2, CD004721

68  Van den Hount, W.B., Van der Linden, Y.M., Steenland, E., Wiggenraad, R.G., Kievit, J., de Haes, H., and Leer, J.W. (2003). Single-versus multiple-fraction radiotherapy in patients with painful bone metastases: cost-utility analysis based on a randomized trial. *J Natl Cancer Inst*, 95, 222–229.

69  Weinberger, B. (2000). Overcoming the obstacles of pain management. In *Annual Congress-Symposia highlights*, pp.13–14. Expert panel held at the Oncology Nursing Society Annual Congress, San Antonio, TX.

70  Sapienza, M.T., Ono, C.R., Guimaraes, M.I., Watanabe, T., Costa, P.A., and Buchpiguel, C.A. (2004). Retrospective evaluation of bone pain palliation after samarium-153-EDTMP therapy. *Rev Hosp Clin Fac Med Sao Paulo*, 59, 321–328.

71  Roqué, M., Martinez, M.J., Alonso-Coello, P., Catalá, E., García, J.L., and Ferrandiz, M. (2003). Radioisotopes for metastatic bone pain. *Cochrane Database Syst Rev*, 4, CD003347.

72  Coleman, R.E. (1997). Skeletal complications of malignancy. *Cancer*, 80 (Suppl. 8), 1588–1594.

73  Brown, J.E., Neville-Webbe, H., and Coleman, R.E. (2004). The role of bisphosphonates in breast and prostate cancers. *Endocrine-Related Cancer*, 11, 207–224.

74 Rogers, M.J., Watts, D.J., and Russell, R.G. (1997). Overview of bisphosphonates. *Cancer*, 80, 1652–1660.

75 Body, J.J., Bartl, R., Burckhardt, P., and Delmas, P.D. (1998). Current use of bisphosphonates in oncology. *J Clin Oncol*, 16, 3890–3899.

76 Pavlakis, N. and Stockler, M. (2004). Bisphosphonates for breast cancer (Cochrane review). *Cochrane Database Syst Rev*, 3, CD 003474.

77 Wong, R. and Wiffen, P.J. (2002). Bisphosphonates for the relief of pain secondary to bone metastases. *Cochrane Database syst Rev.*, 2., CD 002068.

78 Kristensen, B., Ejlertsen, B., Groenvold, M., Hein, S., and Loft, H. (1999). Oral clodronate in breast cancer patients with bone metastases: a randomized study. *J Int Med*, 246, 67–74

79 Theriault, R.L., *et al.* (1999). Pamidronate reduces skeletal morbidity in women with advance breast cancer and lytic bone lesions: a randomized placebo-controlled trial. *J Clin Oncol*, 17, 846–854.

80 Body, J.J., Lichinitser, M.R., and Diehl, I.E. (1999). Double-blind placebo controlled trial of ibandronate in breast cancer metastatic bone. *Proceed Am Soc Clin Oncol*, 18, 575a.

81 Rosen, L.S., Gordon, D., Kaminsi, M., Howell, A., Belch, A., *et al.* (2001). Zoledronic acid versus pamidronate in the treatment of skeletal metastases in patients with breast cancer or osteolytic lesions of multiple myeloma; a phase II, double-blind, comparative trial. *Cancer J*, 7, 337–387.

82 Jensen, M., Evans, A., Mathis, J., Kallmes, D., Cloft, H., and Dion, J. (1997). Percutaneous polymethylmethacrilate vertebroplasty in the treatment of osteopororotic vertebral body compression fractures: technical aspects. AJNR *Am J Neuroradiol*, 18, 1897–1904.

83 Diamond, T., Champion, B., and Clark, W. (2003). Management of acute osteoporotic vertebral fractures a nonrandomized trial comparing percutaneous vertebroplasty with conservative therapy. *Am J Med*, 114, 257–265.

84 Lieberman, I. and Reinhardt, M.K. (2003). Vertebroplasty and kyphoplasty for osteolytic vertebrae collapse. *Clin Orthopedics Related Res*, 415, 176–186.

85 Neeman, Z. and Wood, B.J. (2002). Radiofrequency ablation beyond the liver. *Techniques Vascular Interventional Radiol*, 5, 156–163.

86 Goetz, M.P., Callstrom, M.R., Charboneau, W., *et al.* (2004). Percutaneous image-guided radiofrequency ablation of painful metastases involving bone. A multicenter study. *J Clin Oncol*, 22, 300–306.

87 Struthers, C., Mayer, D., and Fisher, G. (1998). Nursing management of the patient with bone metastases. *Sem Oncol Nursing*, 14, 199–209.

88 Grill, V., Rankin, W., and Martin, T.J. (1998). Parathyroid hormone-related protein (PTHrP) and hypercalcemia. *Eur J Cancer*, 34, 222–229.

89 Twycross, R. (1997). Biochemical syndromes. In Twycross, R., ed. *Symptom management in advanced cancer*, pp. 132–142. Oxford, Radcliffe Medical Press.

90 Ralston, S.H., Fogelman, I., Gardner, M.D., and Boyle, I.T. (1984). Relative contribution of humoral and metastatic factors to the pathogenesis of hypercalcaemia of malignancy. *BMJ*, 288, 1405–1408.

91 Wimalawansa, S.J. (1994). Significance of plasma PTH-rP in patients with hypercalcaemia of malignancy treated with bisphosphonate. *Cancer*, 73, 2223–2230.

92 Bajorunas, D.R. (1990). Clinical manifestations of cancer related hypercalcaemia. *Semin Oncol*, 17 (Suppl. 5), 16–25.

93 Bilezikian, J.P. (1992). Management of acute hypercalcaemia. *N Engl J Med*, 326, 1196–1203.

94 Khristensen, B., Ejlertsen, B., Mouridsen, H.T., and Loft, H. (1998). Survival in breast cancer patients after the first episode of hypercalcaemia. *J Inten Med*, **244**, 189–198.

95 Ross, J.R., Saunders, Y., Edmonds, P.M., Patel, S., Wonderling, D., Normand, C., *et al*. (2004). A systematic review of the role of bisphosphonates in metastatic disease. *Health Technol Assess*, **8**, number 4, 1–176

96 Sim, F.H., Frassica, F.J., and Chao, E.Y.C. (1995). Orthopaedic management using new devices and prostheses. *Clin Orthop Rel*, **312**, 160–172.

97 Fidler, M.W. (1981). Incidence of fracture through metastases in long bones. *Acta Orthop Scand*, **52**, 623–627.

98 DeWald, R.L., Bridwell, K.H., Prodomas, C., and Roots, M.F. (1985). Reconstructive surgery as palliation for metastatic malignancy of spine. *Spine*, **10**, 21.

99 Townsend, P.W., Rosenthal, H.G., Smalley, S.R., *et al*. (1994). Impact of postoperative radiation therapy and other perioperative factors on outcome after orthopedic stabilization of impending fractures due to metastatic disease. *J Clin Oncol*, **12**, 2345–2350.

100 Blamey, R.W., *et al*. (1999). British Association of Surgical Oncology guidelines. The management of metastatic bone disease in the United Kingdom. *Eur J Surg Oncol*, **25**, 3–23.

101 O'Donoghue, D.S., Howell, A., and Walls, J. (1997). Orthopaedic management of structurally significant bone disease in breast cancer metastases. *J Bone Joint Surg (Br)*, **79B** (suppl1), 98.

102 Loblaw, D.A., Laperriere, N.J., and Mackillop, W.J. (2003). A population-based study of malignant spinal cord compression in Ontario. *Clin Oncol*, **15**, 211–217.

103 Byrne, T.N. (1992). Spinal cord compression from epidural metastases. *N Engl J Med*, **327**, 614–619.

104 Gerstein, P.C. and Welch, W.C. (2000). Current surgical management of metastatic spinal disease. *Oncol (Huntingt)*, **14**, 1013–1024 [discussion 1024, 1029–1030].

105 Cook, A.M., Lau, T.N., Tomlinson, M.J., *et al*. (1998). Magnetic resonance imaging of the whole spine in suspected malignant spinal cord compression, impact on management. *Clin Oncol*, **10**, 39–43

106 Prasad, D. and Schiff, D. (2005). Malignant spinal-cord compression. *Lancet Oncol*, **6**, 15–24.

107 Loblaw, D.A. and Laperierre, N.J. (1998). Emergency treatment of malignant extradural spinal cord compression: an evidence-based guideline. *J Clin Oncol*, **16**, 1613–1624.

108 Abraham, J.L. (1999). Management of pain and spinal cord compression in patients with advanced cancer. *Ann Intern Med*, **131**, 37–47.

109 Siegal, T. (1989). Current considerations in the management of neoplasic spinal cord compression. *Spine*, **14**, 223–228.

110 Sorensen, S., Helweg-Larsen, S., Mouridsen, H., and Hansen, H.H. (1994). Effect of high-dose dexamethasone in carcinomatous metastatic spinal cord compression treated with radiotherapy: a randomised trial. *Eur J Cancer*, **30A**, 22–27.

111 Heimdal, K., Hirschberg, H., Slettebo, H., Watne, K., and Nome, O. (1977). High incidence of serious side effects of high-dose dexamethasone treatment in patients with epidural spinal cord compression. *J Neurosurg*, **47**, 653–658.

112 Pinover, W.H. and Coia, L.R. (1998). Palliative radiation therapy. In Berger, A.M., Porteroy, R.K., and Weissman, D.E., eds. *Principles and practice supportive oncology*, pp. 603–626. Philadelphia, Lippincott-Raven.

113 Maranzano, E. and Latini, P. (1995). Effectiveness of radiation therapy without surgery in metastatic spinal cord compression: final results from prospective trial. *Int J Radiat Oncol Biol Phys*, **32**, 959–967.

114 Cobb, C.A., Leavens, M.E., and Eckles, N. (1977). Indications for nonoperative treatment of spinal cord compression due to breast cancer. *J Neurosurg*, **47**, 653–658.

115 Young, R.F., Post, E.M., and King, G.A. (1980). Treatment of spinal epidural metastases. Randomized prospective comparison of laminectomy and radiotherapy. *J Neurosurg*, **53**, 741–748.

116. Patchell, R., Tibbs, P., and Regine, W. (2003). A randomized trial of direct decompressive surgical resection in the treatment of spinal cord compression caused by metastases. *J Clin Oncol*, **21**, 237.

117 Klimo, P. and Schimidt, M.H. (2004). Surgical management of spinal metastases. *Oncologist*, **9**, 188–196.

118 Green, J.R., Müller, K., and Jaeggi, K.A. (1994). Preclinical pharmacology of CGP 42′446, a new, potent, heterocyclic bisphosphonate compound. *J Bone Miner Res*, **9**, 745–751.

119 Hillner, B.E., Ingle, J.N., Chelebowski, R.T., *et al.* (2003). American Society of Clinical Oncology 2003 update on the role of bisphosphonates and bone health issues in women with breast cancer. *J Clin Oncol*, **21**, 4042–4057.

120 Coleman, R.E. (2004). Bisphosphonates: clinical experience. *Oncologist*, **9** (Suppl. 4), 14–27.

121 Baines, M.J. (2002). Spinal cord compression – a personal and palliative care perspective. *Clin Oncol*, **14**, 135–138.

122 Levack, P., Graham, J., Collie, D., Grant, R., Kidd, J., Kunkler, I., Gibson, A., Hurman, D., McMillan, N., Rampling, R., Slider, L., Statham, P., and Summers, D. (2002). The Scottish Cord Compression Study Group. *Clin Oncol*, **14**, 472–480.

Chapter 10

# The management of malignant pleural effusions in breast cancer

Scott A. North, Anil A. Joy, and John R. Mackey

## Introduction

Malignant pleural effusions are one of the most common problems that face women with advanced breast cancer. Breast cancer is the second leading cause of malignant pleural effusions. Historically, nearly 50% of women with metastatic breast cancer develop pleural effusions at some point in their disease trajectory,[1] and autopsy series have identified pleural metastases in up to 65% of women dying from breast cancer.[2] Although the interval from initial breast cancer diagnosis to recognition of pleural metastases is variable, pleural metastases are usually an indication of widespread systemic disease, and pleural metastases as the only sign of recurrence is relatively rare.[3] The median survival after diagnosis of pleural metastases is highly variable, but improvements in systemic breast cancer therapy are now giving modest increases in the overall duration of survival in women with metastatic breast cancer (see Chapter 1).[4–6] Nonetheless, pleural effusions remain a major problem for women with advanced breast cancer, and effective palliation of pleural effusions can greatly improve quality of life.

## Pathophysiology
### The normal physiology of pleural fluid

The pleural space is the area located between the visceral pleura (the surface lining the outside of each lung) and the parietal pleura (the surface lining the inside of the chest wall) and is lined by mesothelial cells. This space normally contains up to 20 ml of fluid which acts as a lubricant to facilitate the movement of the lungs and chest wall during respiration. The composition of normal pleural fluid is similar to that of plasma, except that the protein concentration is below 20 g/l. In the normal setting, the pleural fluid is produced by hydrostatic pressure from the parietal pleura (with lesser amounts generated from the visceral pleura) and is reabsorbed primarily by lymphatic channels between the mesothelial cells of the parietal pleura. The visceral pleura plays a relatively small role in pleural fluid turnover under normal physiological conditions.[7]

### Routes of metastasis

The routes followed by breast cancer cells metastasizing to the pleura are still a matter of debate. Although direct tumour extension can produce pleural effusions, the majority of pleural metastases are thought to arise from dissemination via haematogenous and lymphatic spread. In an overview of eight reports including nearly 500 breast cancer patients, effusions were ipsilateral to the original breast cancer in 62% of cases, contralateral in 25%, and bilateral in 13%.[8]

## Mechanisms of pleural fluid accumulation

In general, effusions are directly related to serosal involvement with metastatic deposits. Once metastases are established in the pleural surface, several processes may contribute to the abnormal accumulation of fluid. Increased capillary vascular permeability and leakages plays a principal role in the development of the exudative pleural effusions typically seen with advanced breast cancer. The critical factor appears to be vascular endothelial growth factor (VEGF), a potent endothelial cell-specific mitogen that promotes angiogenesis, vascular hyperpermeability, and vasodilatation by autocrine mechanisms involving nitric oxide. In patients with malignant pleural effusions, VEGF levels were noted to be significantly higher than those seen in other causes of pleural effusion[9,10] – the cutoff of 2000 pg/ml was proposed as a highly sensitive indicator of malignant effusion.[10] VEGF levels have also been noted to be substantially higher in haemorrhagic pleural effusions as opposed to non-haemorrhagic effusions.[11] In *in vitro* and animal models of malignant pleural effusions, strategies to antagonize the VEGF activity and its signalling pathway have shown some success.[12] Advanced breast cancer clinical trials with anti-VEGF drugs are currently ongoing, so the efficacy of these agents on pleural effusions will soon be known.

Additionally, pleural effusions can also occur in women with advanced breast cancer other than directly mediated by pleural metastasis. Lymphangitic carcinomatosis of the lungs and extensive hilar or mediastinal lymph node deposits can impair visceral lymphatic drainage. Severe hypoalbuminaemia can occur in advanced cancer states, which results in a subsequent decrease in vascular oncotic pressure, inducing the formation of pleural effusions, as well.

Health-care providers must also be aware that several non-cancer-related causes of pleural effusions also exist, making it important to document the cause of an effusion before ascribing it to metastatic disease. Congestive heart failure, a complication of some breast cancer therapies including anthracyclines, trastuzumab, and cardiac radiation, can increase hydrostatic pressure and lead to pleural fluid accumulation. Pneumonia and pulmonary emboli occur commonly in women with advanced breast cancer, and can cause exudative non-malignant effusions. Occasionally, breast cancer treatment itself can trigger a pleural effusion. In one clinical trial of weekly administration of docetaxel, 20% of patients developed drug-related pleural effusions.[13]

## Clinical presentation and diagnosis

Diagnosis and definition of the aetiology of a pleural effusion begins with a careful history, physical examination, and analysis of the pleural fluid. Although approximately one-quarter of patients are asymptomatic at the time of diagnosis, cough is the most common symptom. Dyspnoea on exertion is also frequent, and dyspnoea at rest may be more marked when the patient is lying on the side contralateral to the effusion.

Pleuritic chest pain is uncommon. Physical findings include tachycardia, decreased air entry, and associated dullness to percussion of the affected hemithorax. Although chest radiography will show the location and size of effusions, ultrasonography is very useful to confirm that fluid, and not just pleural thickening and metastases, is present, and it can reliably detect potentially coexisting pericardial effusion.

Malignant pleural effusions can occasionally be the first indication of recurrent breast cancer. In this situation, cytological diagnosis is an essential part of management to confirm the recurrent nature of disease. In the setting of known recurrent or widespread metastatic breast cancer, cytological confirmation of the malignant nature of a pleural effusion is of importance primarily to rule out other, non-malignant, causes of the effusion.

The cornerstone of the diagnosis of malignant effusions is pleural fluid cytology – the presence of malignant cells in the fluid is the only absolutely diagnostic test for malignant pleural effusions. Reported positive cytology rates are variable, in part due to variation in technique and in the populations studied. To optimize the diagnostic yield, we recommend that at least 250 ml of pleural fluid be sent to the laboratory for centrifugation and cytospin examination. If negative, two additional diagnostic thoracentesis can raise the yield to over 80% positivity.[14,15]

In general, the remaining laboratory tests lack sufficient sensitivity, specificity, or predictive accuracy to be definitive for the diagnosis of malignant pleural effusion. For example, although the majority of malignant effusions are exudative (i.e. the pleural fluid:serum protein ratio is greater than 0.5), up to 20% of malignant effusions are transudative. Similarly, pleural fluid evaluation for glucose, pH, carcinoembryonic antigen, and flow cytometry are of limited use in the initial diagnostic evaluation of pleural effusion. However, should three thoracentesis fail to yield malignant cells or infectious agents in an exudative effusion, pleural biopsy has been recommended and can confirm malignancy in up to 50% of cytology-negative cases.[14–16]

# Physical removal of malignant pleural effusions

For most patients with pleural effusions, the physical removal of fluid serves a dual purpose of both diagnostic and therapeutic utility. In patients with asymptomatic effusions receiving systemic therapy, observation alone is a reasonable initial approach. The vast majority of malignant pleural effusions, however, progress and eventually become symptomatic, with only a rare minority achieving a steady state balance of fluid production and removal. Palliation is the goal, with relief of symptoms essential, and this can be achieved by a variety of non-surgical and surgical interventions depending on the clinical context and life expectancy of the patient (Fig. 10.1).

## Therapeutic thoracocentesis

Needle thoracocentesis is recommended for the initial relief of dyspnoea and to obtain diagnostic confirmation of malignancy. Caution should be employed when more than 1.5 l is drained in one sitting or if the fluid is removed too quickly, as there is a theoretical risk of re-expansion pulmonary oedema.[17] The procedure should be aborted, at any fluid amount, if intolerable symptoms arise (e.g. dyspnoea, cough,

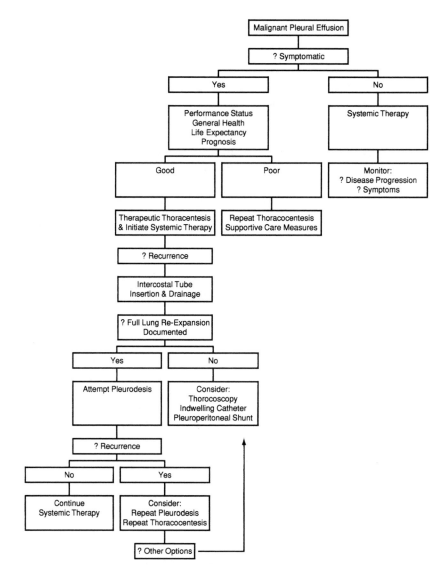

**Fig. 10.1** Management of malignant pleural effusions.

or significant chest discomfort). In selected patients, such as those with short life expectancy or severe debilitation, repeat needle thoracocentesis can be undertaken. For all others cases, a more definitive method of fluid removal should be sought, as the risk of recurrence after pleural aspiration alone is exceedingly high.

## Intercostal tube insertion and drainage

Intercostal tube insertion is the most commonly employed and cost-effective method of pleural fluid drainage. Similar success rates have been reported with either large

(24–32 French) or small (10–14 French) bore tubes, with the latter offering more in the way of comfort with no significant difference in tube blockage or effusion control success rates.[18–20]

A variety of sclerosing agents are available for instillation with the effectiveness of each discussed in detail below. Prior to performing pleurodesis, pleural fluid should be drained in a controlled fashion with demonstrated symptom relief and full lung re-expansion documented radiologically. Full lung re-expansion brings the visceral and parietal pleural surfaces in contact with one another and allows the sclerosant to fuse the two surfaces, obliterating the potential space and thus preventing reaccumulation of the malignant fluid.

In a randomized study that compared short-term versus long-term tube thoracostomy drainage, the standard recommendation of obtaining <150 ml/day drainage was less important than documenting full lung re-expansion prior to tetracycline pleurodesis.[21] Attempting pleurodesis in cases where trapped lung or bronchial obstruction is suspected is less efficacious; however, it can be considered in cases where the patient is poorly suited for other surgical interventions.

In the absence of excessive fluid drainage (>250 ml/day), the intercostal tube should be removed within 12–72 h of sclerosant instillation. In cases where excessive fluid drainage persists, repeat pleurodesis may be attempted with an alternative sclerosant. In cases of non-reversible incomplete lung expansion, the tube may be removed as pleurodesis is unlikely to succeed. The role of intrapleural fibrinolysis should only be considered in cases of symptomatic multiloculated effusions resistant to simple drainage, as the evidence for this procedure is quite limited.[22,23]

## Indwelling catheter drainage

In certain circumstances, symptomatic recurrent malignant pleural effusions can be effectively controlled by long-term indwelling catheter drainage. This procedure also has the advantage of being particularly useful in cases where trapped lung is identified. Small-bore pig-tail catheter insertion can be performed blinded or via ultrasonographic guidance with demonstrated efficacy in symptomatic relief of dyspnea.[24,25] Specifically designed long-term tunnelled pleural catheters (e.g. Pleurx$^®$) are a relatively new treatment option, allowing patients to be treated on an outpatient basis. With the indwelling catheter in place, the patient, trained family members, or knowledgeable health-care providers can drain pleural effusions intermittently at home. When compared with doxycycline pleurodesis via tube thoracostomy, the tunnelled pleural catheter required shorter hospitalization, could be managed on an outpatient basis, and was deemed to be cost-effective.[26,27] Catheter insertion requires specially trained personnel and appropriate follow-up facilities need to be in place when outpatient management is considered.

## Thoracoscopic management

Thoracoscopy can be performed under local, regional, or general anaesthesia and allows for direct visualization of intrathoracic structures and biopsy of any suspicious parietal lesions. In selected circumstances, it can also be used for therapeutic means, as in the case of mechanical lysis of adhesions in multiloculated malignant pleural effusions. Talc poudrage and chest tube insertion for pleurodesis can also be performed effectively in this manner.

## Thoracotomy approach

Thoracotomy is occasionally required in the management of refractory recurrent malignant pleural effusions. Pleural abrasion, with or without parietal pleurectomy, can be performed via formal thoracotomy or via video assisted thoracic surgery (VATS). Pleurectomy involves the physical removal of the parietal pleura, along with any associated disease from the chest wall. As an invasive procedure it carries an increased risk of morbidity (e.g. haemorrhage and infection), in addition to operative mortality.[28,29] These potential risks emphasize the importance of careful patient selection if this aggressive approach is undertaken.

## Pleuroperitoneal shunt

Pleuroperitoneal shunting can be attempted in those individuals with intractable, recurrent pleural effusions who are unable to tolerate a large surgical procedure. The shunt is a valved chamber which is inserted across the diaphragm, with fenestrated pleural and peritoneal catheters attached at either end. The device can be inserted via thoracoscopy or a thoracotomy approach. The malignant fluid flows from the pleural space to the peritoneal cavity, either via pressure gradient or via manual pumping. Effective control of malignant pleural effusions in cases of trapped lung can also be achieved.[30,31] The device should not be inserted in cases where multiple loculations are identified, if known empyema is present, or if the patient is unable to manually pump the apparatus for whatever reason.

# Pharmacological management of malignant effusions

Pharmacological management of malignant pleural effusions in the breast cancer patient can consist of systemic management of the cancer, local treatment of the effusion itself, or a combination of both. Treatment decisions are guided by the severity and rapidity of onset of the effusion, prior exposure of the patient to antineoplastic therapy, and the patient's performance status.

## Systemic anticancer treatment

Because malignant pleural effusions are typically due to the presence of breast cancer in the pleural space, systemic anticancer therapy can result in regression of the tumour and resolution of the effusion. Breast cancer is frequently responsive to both chemotherapy and hormonal treatment, the details of which are beyond the scope of this review. Systemic management alone is typically employed in patients with small volume effusions who are minimally symptomatic. Since pleural metastases are seldom the only site of metastatic disease, chemotherapy or hormonal therapy is generally indicated for the overall management of metastatic disease in addition to the pleural effusion.

## Local pharmacological management

Local pharmacological management of a pleural effusion consists of complete drainage of the pleural fluid, usually by chest tube insertion, and instillation of various agents into the pleural space in the hope that they will cause a sclerosing reaction that obliterates the pleural space, thus preventing fluid reaccumulation. The efficacy of these agents tends to be dependent on maximal drainage of the pleural fluid in order to ensure good contact of the sclerosant with the pleural surface and to avoid dilution of the drug being used. Agents commonly instilled into the pleural space to induce sclerosis include chemotherapeutic agents, antibiotics, steroids, and talc.

### Chemotherapeutic agents

Chemotherapy instillation into the pleural space is performed with the intent that there will be both an antineoplastic effect from the agent being used and that the agent will act as a sclerosant, inciting intense pleural irritation. Several chemotherapeutic agents have been tried, including mechlorethamine, cisplatin, cytarabine, mitoxantrone,[32] and bleomycin. In general, trials have been performed in patients with diverse malignancies, and results restricted to breast-cancer-related effusions are not reported. Of the chemotherapeutic agents, bleomycin has been most widely studied and compared to other agents. In one series, 69% of patients had no recurrence of their pleural effusion 30 days after bleomycin instillation following complete drainage of their effusion via chest tube.[33] This compares favourably with other sclerosing agents and is superior to other chemotherapeutic agents that have been used for effusion management. The major drawbacks to bleomycin are related to the systemic inflammatory response that may be seen, such as fever, chills, and local pain after instillation, and drug acquisition cost.[34] In addition, there are concerns about drug absorption and toxicity from the chemotherapy itself, as well as safe handling of the cytotoxic agent. Several studies have compared bleomycin to talc pleurodesis and have found talc to be either equivalent or superior to bleomycin.[34–38] This has led to a preference to use talc and, thus, bleomycin instillation is rarely performed.

### Antibiotics

The two most widely studied agents in this class are tetracycline and doxycycline. Complete response rates to tetracycline use range from 15–69% in various series. Several studies have compared bleomycin (considered to be the best chemotherapeutic sclerosing agent) to tetracycline.[38–40] In all of these, tetracycline was either equivalent or inferior to bleomycin with respect to effusion control at 30 days post-treatment, as well as median time to reaccumulation of the effusion. When compared to talc pleurodesis, tetracycline is an inferior agent (see below). Tetracycline has also been criticized as it usually requires multiple instillations, which extends hospitalization and thus drives up health-care costs. Since the early 1990s a formulation suitable for intrapleural use has not been commercially available in many countries.

Doxycycline has also been compared to bleomycin in controlling malignant effusions. In one randomized study, 23/29 (79%) patients instilled with doxycycline had not recurred by the 30 day mark, a result not statistically different from bleomycin-treated patients.[18] Doxycycline used in combination with *Corynebacterium parvum* has also demonstrated response rates of around 75%.[41] Major drawbacks to doxycycline are that, again, many patients require repeated instillations, which prolongs hospitalization. In addition, 50% of patients develop pain and fever post instillation.

## Talc

Talc instillation causes an intense pleuritis and is believed by many to be the best sclerosant available for management of malignant pleural effusions, with complete response rates as high as 90%. Unlike antibiotics or antineoplastic agents, talc is not cleared form the pleural space and this may contribute to its effectiveness.

It is felt that uniform distribution of talc over the entire pleural surface is important in obtaining a good result. This has led to various methods of instilling the talc, including the creation of a talc slurry that is instilled via a chest tube at bedside as well as video-assisted thoracoscopy done under general anaesthesia with insufflation of dry powder. Patients with malignant effusions often have poor performance status and compromised lung function, making general anaesthesia and extensive operative procedures undesirable. A randomized study was undertaken to determine if either of these techniques was more effective.[42] It was found that talc slurry was equally effective to direct insufflation of talc during thoracoscopy in achieving complete effusion control. This has led to bedside talc slurry instillation as the preferred method of administering this agent.

Talc has been compared to chemotherapeutic agents, most commonly bleomycin, in terms of effusion control. In one study, 90% of patients treated with talc via bedside thoracostomy had complete resolution of their effusion as compared to 79% of bleomycin-treated patients, a statistically significant result.[34] This result was confirmed by another group of investigators who demonstrated 89% of patients treated with a talc slurry as compared to 70% of bleomycin-treated patients achieved complete response.[35] Talc is also considerably less expensive than bleomycin and has fewer problems related to chest pain or systemic reactions after instillation.

When compared to tetracycline, talc also demonstrates favourable results. In one randomized trial of talc insufflation vs. either bleomycin or tetracycline instillation, only 33% of tetracycline-treated patients had effusion control at 30 days compared to 97% of talc-treated patients.[38]

Based on the best current available literature, talc appears to be the preferred agent to instill into the pleural space to effect a pleurodesis. It is safe to administer at the bedside as a talc slurry after chest tube drainage of the effusion and is highly effective in achieving pleurodesis, doing so on average in 90% of treated patients. It is also a very cost effective agent compared to other readily available sclerosants and is well tolerated by patients with low rates of pain (5–10%) and systemic febrile reactions (15–20%).

## Glucocorticosteroids

Several investigators have examined the role of steroid instillation for the management of malignant effusions such as pleural effusion and malignant ascites. Mackey *et al.* demonstrated that steroid instillation after therapeutic paracentesis delayed time to recurrence of the ascites and improved patient self-reported quality of life.[43] Bartal performed a small phase II non-randomized trial of intrapleural steroid instillation in breast cancer patients after therapeutic thoracentesis.[44] In that study, 6/10 patients had symptomatic benefit and 3/10 patients had complete resolution of their effusion. A randomized phase III study comparing instillation of methylprednisolone acetate versus placebo post-thoracentesis was performed by North *et al.* to confirm these results.[45] Sixty-seven patients were enrolled on study, of which 65% were breast cancer patients. The results showed that there was no improvement in quality of life or time to recurrence of pleural effusions for steroid-treated patients as compared to those receiving placebo injections. Thus, steroid instillation should not be considered a useful strategy to manage these patients.

## Conclusion

Malignant pleural effusion is a common and serious complication of advanced breast cancer. Although responsive to a variety of pharmacological therapies and surgical interventions, appropriately selecting treatments to palliate the accompanying cough and dyspnoea requires good clinical judgement. Therapeutic choices based on the patient's symptoms, performance status, and degree of prior exposure to systemic therapies for breast cancer are most likely to minimize hospitalization time, improvement of symptoms, and preserve quality of life.

## References

1  Fracchia, A.A., Knapper, W.H., Carey, J.T., and Farrow, J.H. (1970). Intrapleural chemotherapy for effusion from metastatic breast carcinoma. *Cancer*, 26, 626–629.

2  Abrams, H.C. (1950). Metastases in carcinoma: Analysis of 1000 autopsied cases. *Cancer*, 3, 74–85.

3  Kamby, C., Vejborg, I., Kristensen, B., Olsen, L.O., and Mouridsen, H.T. (1988). Metastatic pattern in recurrent breast cancer. Special reference to intrathoracic recurrences. *Cancer*, 62, 2226–2233.

4  Nabholtz, J.M., Senn, H.J., Bezwoda, W.R., Melnychuk, D., Deschenes, L., Douma, J., *et al.* (1999). Prospective randomized trial of docetaxel versus mitomycin plus vinblastine in patients with metastatic breast cancer progressing despite previous anthracycline-containing chemotherapy. 304 Study Group. *J Clin Oncol*, 17, 1413–1424.

5  Slamon, D.J., Leyland-Jones, B., Shak, S., Fuchs, H., Paton, V., Bajamonde, A., *et al.* (2001). Use of chemotherapy plus a monoclonal antibody against HER2 for metastatic breast cancer that overexpresses HER2. *NEJM*, 344, 783–792.

6  O'Shaughnessy, J., Miles, D., Vukelja, S., Moiseyenko, V., Ayoub, J.P., Cervantes, G., *et al.* (2002). Superior survival with capecitabine plus docetaxel combination therapy in anthracycline-pretreated patients with advanced breast cancer: phase III trial results. *J Clin Oncol*, 20, 2812–2823.

7  Miserocchi, G. (1997). Physiology and pathophysiology of pleural fluid turnover. *Eur Respir J*, 10, 219–225.

8  Johnson, K.A., Kramer, B.S., and Crane, J.M. (1998). Management of pleural metastases in breast cancer. In Bland, K.I. and Copeland, E.M., eds. *The breast: comprehensive management of benign and malignant diseases*, 2nd edn. Philadelphia, W.B. Saunders.

9 Hamed, E.A., El-Noweihi, A.M., Mohamed, A.Z., and Mahmoud, A. (2004). Vasoactive mediators (VEGF and TNF-alpha) in patients with malignant and tuberculous pleural effusions. *Respirology*, **9**, 81–86.

10 Momi, H., Matsuyama, W., Inoue, K., Kawabata, M., Arimura, K., Fukunaga, H., *et al.* (2002). Vascular endothelial growth factor and proinflammatory cytokines in pleural effusions. *Respir Med*, **96**, 817–822.

11 Ishimoto, O., Saijo, Y., Narumi, K., Kimura, Y., Ebina, M., Matsubara, N., *et al.* (2002). High level of vascular endothelial growth factor in hemorrhagic pleural effusion of cancer. *Oncology*, **63**, 70–75.

12 Grove, C.S. and Lee, Y.C. (2002). Vascular endothelial growth factor: the key mediator in pleural effusion formation. *Curr Opin Pulm Med*, **8**, 294–301.

13 Kuroi, K., Bando, H., Saji, S., and Toi, M. (2003). Protracted administration of weekly docetaxel in metastatic breast cancer. *Oncol Rep*, **10**, 1479–1484.

14 Salyer, W.R., Eggleston, J.C., and Erozan, Y.S. (1975). Efficacy of pleural needle biopsy and pleural fluid cytopathology in the diagnosis of malignant neoplasm involving the pleura. *Chest*, **67**, 536–539.

15 Prakash, U.B. and Reiman, H.M. (1985). Comparison of needle biopsy with cytologic analysis for the evaluation of pleural effusion: analysis of 414 cases. *Mayo Clin Proc*, **60**, 158–164.

16 Al-Shimemeri, A.A., Al-Ghadeer, H.M., and Giridhar, H.R. (2003). Diagnostic yield of closed pleural biopsy in exudative pleural effusion. *Saudi Med J*, **24**, 282–286.

17 Tarver, R.D., Broderick, L.S., and Conces, D.J., Jr. (1996). Reexpansion pulmonary edema. *J Thorac Imaging*, **11**, 198–209.

18 Patz, E.F.J., McAdams, H.P., Erasmus, J.J., Goodman, P.C., Culhane, D.K., Gilkeson, R.C., *et al.* (1998). Sclerotherapy for malignant pleural effusions: a prospective randomized trial of bleomycin vs doxycycline with small-bore catheter drainage. *Chest*, **113**, 1305–1311.

19 Clementsen, P., Evald, T., Grode, G., Hansen, M., Krag Jacobsen, G., and Faurschou, P. (1998). Treatment of malignant pleural effusion: pleurodesis using a small percutaneous catheter. A prospective randomized study. *Respir Med*, **92**, 593–596.

20 Parulekar, W., Di Primio, G., Matzinger, F., Dennie, C., and Bociek, G. (2001). Use of small-bore vs large-bore chest tubes for treatment of malignant pleural effusions. *Chest*, **120**, 19–25.

21 Villanueva, A.G., Gray, A.W., Jr., Shahian, D.M., Williamson, W.A., and Beamis, J.F., Jr. (1994). Efficacy of short term versus long term tube thoracostomy drainage before tetracycline pleurodesis in the treatment of malignant pleural effusions. *Thorax*, **49**, 23–25.

22 Davies, C.W., Traill, Z.C., Gleeson, F.V., and Davies, R.J. (1999). Intrapleural streptokinase in the management of malignant multiloculated pleural effusions. *Chest*, **115**, 729–733.

23 Gilkeson, R.C., Silverman, P., and Haaga, J.R. (1999). Using urokinase to treat malignant pleural effusions. AJR. *Am J Roentgenol*, **173**, 781–783.

24 Chen, Y.M., Shih, J.F., Yang, K.Y., Lee, Y.C., and Perng, R.P. (2000). Usefulness of pig-tail catheter for palliative drainage of malignant pleural effusions in cancer patients. *Support Care Cancer*, **8**, 423–426.

25 Chella, A., Ribechini, A., Dini, P., Adamo, C., Mussi, A., and Angeletti, C.A. (1994). [Treatment of malignant pleural effusion by percutaneous catheter drainage and chemical pleurodesis]. *Minerva Chir*, **49**, 1077–1082.

26 Putnam, J.B., Jr., Light, R.W., Rodriguez, R.M., Ponn, R., Olak, J., Pollak, J.S., *et al.* (1999). A randomized comparison of indwelling pleural catheter and doxycycline pleurodesis in the management of malignant pleural effusions. *Cancer*, **86**, 1992–1999.

27 Putnam, J.B., Jr., Walsh, G.L., Swisher, S.G., Roth, J.A., Suell, D.M., Vaporciyan, A.A., *et al.* (2000). Outpatient management of malignant pleural effusion by a chronic indwelling pleural catheter. *Ann Thorac Surg,* 69, 369–375.

28 Martini, N., Bains, M.S., and Beattie, E.J., Jr. (1975). Indications for pleurectomy in malignant effusion. *Cancer,* 35, 734–738.

29 Fry, W.A. and Khandekar, J.D. (1995). Parietal pleurectomy for malignant pleural effusion. *Ann Surg Oncol,* 2, 160–164.

30 Petrou, M., Kaplan, D., and Goldstraw, P. (1995). Management of recurrent malignant pleural effusions. The complementary role of talc pleurodesis and pleuroperitoneal shunting. *Cancer,* 75, 801–805.

31 Genc, O., Petrou, M., Ladas, G., and Goldstraw, P. (2000). The long-term morbidity of pleuroperitoneal shunts in the management of recurrent malignant effusions. Eur J *Cardiothorac Surg,* 18, 143–146.

32 Barbetakis, N., Antoniadis, T., and Tsilikas, C. (2004). Results of chemical pleurodesis with mitoxantrone in malignant pleural effusion from breast cancer. *World J Surg Oncol,* 2, 16.

33 Ostrowski, M.J. (1986). An assessment of the long-term results of controlling reaccumulation of malignant effusions using intracavity bleomycin. *Cancer,* 57, 721.

34 Zimmer, P.W., Hill, M., Casey, K., Harvey, E., and Low, D.E. (1997). Prospective randomized trial of talc slurry vs bleomycin in pleurodesis for symptomatic malignant pleural effusions. *Chest,* 112, 430–434.

35 Ong, K.C., Indumathi, V., Raghuram, J., and Ong, Y.Y. (2000). A comparative study of pleurodesis using talc slurry and bleomycin in the management of malignant pleural effusions. *Respirology,* 5, 99–103.

36 Diacon, A.H., Wyser, C., Bolliger, C.T., Tamm, M., Pless, M., Perruchoud, A.P., *et al.* (2000). Prospective randomized comparison of thoracoscopic talc poudrage under local anesthesia versus bleomycin instillation for pleurodesis in malignant pleural effusions. *Am J Respir Critical Care Med,* 162, 1445–1449.

37 Noppen, M., Degreve, J., Mignolet, M., and Vincken, W. (1997). A prospective, randomized study comparing the efficacy of talc slurry and bleomycin in the treatment of malignant pleural effusions. *Acta Clinica Belgica,* 52, 258–262.

38 Martinez-Moragon, E., Aparicio, J., Rogado, M.C., Sanchis, J., Sanchis, F., and Gil-Suay, V. (1997). Pleurodesis in malignant pleural effusions: a randomized study of tetracycline versus bleomycin. *Eur Respir J,* 10, 2380–2383.

39 Emad, A. and Rezaian, G.R. (1996). Treatment of malignant pleural effusions with a combination of bleomycin and tetracycline. A comparison of bleomycin or tetracycline alone versus a combination of bleomycin and tetracycline. *Cancer,* 78, 2498–2501.

40 Moffett, M.J. and Ruckdeschel, J.C. (1992). Bleomycin and tetracycline in malignant pleural effusions: a review. *Semin Oncol,* 19, 59–62.

41 Salomaa, E.R., Pulkki, K., and Helenius, H. (1995). Pleurodesis with doxycycline or Corynebacterium parvum in malignant pleural effusion. *Acta Oncolog,* 34, 117–121.

42 Yim, A.P., Chan, A.T., Lee, T.W., Wan, I.Y., and Ho, J.K. (1996). Thoracoscopic talc insufflation versus talc slurry for symptomatic malignant pleural effusion. *Ann Thoracic Surg,* 62, 1655–1658.

43 Mackey, J.R., Wood, L., Nabholtz, J.M., Jensen, J., and Venner, P. (2000). A phase II trial of triamcinolone hexacetanide for symptomatic recurrent malignant ascites. *J Pain Symp Manag,* 19, 193–199.

44 Bartal, A.H., Gazitt, Y., Zidan, G., Vermeul, B., and Robinson, E. (1991). Clinical and flow cytometry characteristics of malignant pleural effusions in patients after intracavitary administration of methylprednisolone acetate. *Cancer*, 67, 3136–3140.

45 North, S.A., Au, H.-J., Halls, S.B., Tkachuk, L., and Mackey, J.R. (2003). A randomized, phase III, double-blind, placebo-controlled trial of intrapleural instillation of methylprednisolone acetate in the management of malignant pleural effusion. *Chest*, 123, 822–827.

# Index